PRECEPTORSHIPS
IN
NURSING
STAFF
DEVELOPMENT

Kathryn L. Morrow, B.S.N., M.S.N.
Providence Hospital
Everett, Washington

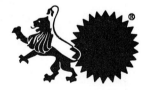

AN ASPEN PUBLICATION®
Aspen Systems Corporation
Rockville, Maryland
Royal Tunbridge Wells
1984

Library of Congress Cataloging in Publication Data

Morrow, Kathryn L.
Preceptorships in nursing staff development.

"An Aspen publication."
Bibliography: p. 265
Includes index.
1. Nursing — Study and teaching (Preceptorship) I. Title. [DNLM:
1. Education, Nursing. 2. Preceptorship. WY 18.5 M883p]
RT74.7.M67   1984   362.1'73'0683   84-6346
ISBN: 0-89443-858-1

Publisher: John R. Marozsan
Associate Publisher: Jack W. Knowles, Jr.
Editorial Director: N. Darlene Como
Executive Managing Editor: Margot G. Raphael
Managing Editor: M. Eileen Higgins
Editorial Services: Martha Sasser
Printing and Manufacturing: Debbie Collins

Library of Congress Catalog Card Number: 84-6346
ISBN: 0-89443-858-1

Printed in the United States of America

To Steve and Mary Jo

Table of Contents

Acknowledgments

Many people helped to make this book a reality. I would like to express my special thanks to my husband Steve and to Ann Gabrielson, who believed in the book and encouraged me to pursue it; to Kay Metters, who helped to type it, and to Dona Martinson, who gave me many helpful suggestions. I owe special thanks to Mary Jo Selg, who spent so many hours of her own time critiquing and suggesting improvements and who continually supported my efforts. I would also like to express my appreciation to Providence Hospital, Everett, Washington, for its support, and to the numerous publishers and authors who so kindly granted me permission to use their materials.

Preface

I became interested in writing this book when I was searching for a similar reference and could find none. Nursing as a profession must take the responsibility to develop new practitioners and I believe the preceptor method to be an ideal way to do this. Although many have advocated use of preceptor programs, few seem to offer detailed practical help. This book, therefore, attempts to provide the practical how-tos of running a preceptor program—how to decide you want one, how to set it up, run it, develop it, and above all how to work with preceptors to accomplish the program's objectives. I do not pretend to have all the answers and hope that this book will spur others to share their experiences and techniques.

Although I attempt to be reasonably comprehensive, so much information exists that is applicable to preceptors that to be totally so is nearly impossible. Therefore, if I have skipped information that seems to be essential, it was not from disinterest but from oversight. Many times I have taken the middle road and have included information in its briefer forms rather than dwelling expansively on it. The bibliography and selected references are meant to supplement this briefness.

Preceptorships in Nursing Staff Development is divided into three sections: a general overview of preceptors, how they can be utilized and the benefits they offer; a section on program development; and a section on preceptor development. The final section, divided into chapters on communication, supervision, adult learners, and the like is meant to serve two purposes: to give the basics of such information to anyone who needs to review them and to offer such information in a compiled form to people working with preceptors. One of my greatest frustrations as I worked with preceptors was the lack of such a reference; each bit of information had to be pulled from its source. While such a search is essential to a scholar, this approach is so time consuming that it is impractical for day-to-day existence. By providing such a reference I hope to save others much of the frustration I myself experienced.

Two notes of explanation: first, the term *head nurse*, used throughout the book, refers to the first line manager of the nursing areas. Although I realize that this term is outdated in many facilities, or has been replaced with titles such as *clinical coordinator*, no one term is standard. Therefore, to minimize confusion only the one title of head nurse has been used.

Second, I have chosen to use the term *novice* throughout the book to refer to the preceptee—the person being precepted. Although a variety of terms are used to describe persons being socialized into new roles or positions, none is comprehensive. *Orientee*, *resident*, and *intern*, for example, have differing connotations. The term *novice* was chosen, for lack of a better one, to encompass all persons being socialized into new roles or positions, as all are novices at the particular role or position. A new graduate nurse, for example, is a novice at both the role of staff nurse and at the position of staff nurse at Hospital X. An experienced nurse, accepting a new position with Hospital X, is not a novice at the position of staff nurse but is still new at the role of staff nurse at Hospital X. I am aware of the difficulties inherent in using such a term and approach but, given the subject, others seemed too limited in their scope.

Working as a preceptor and with preceptors has been a rewarding, albeit at times frustrating, experience. I would not have missed it, nor would I willingly forego it. I wish you the same rewards and hope that this book will prove useful to you in your endeavors.

Kathryn L. Morrow

Part I

Developing and Managing a Preceptor Program

Chapter 1

An Overview of Preceptorship

Nursing today is challenged more than ever before to provide personal, high quality, cost-effective nursing care. This requires that individual nurses accept ever-increasing responsibility for continued personal and professional growth. At the same time, nursing administrators and educators must seek new and innovative ways to develop nursing talent within their institutions. Preceptorship provides one method of assisting current nursing professionals to develop future nursing leaders.

Preceptorship is based on the mentor concept used traditionally in industry and business. Historically, mentorship was the formal or informal relationship that developed between a successful, older, established individual and a younger one. The established person would counsel and support the younger one, assisting him or her to advance in a given business or professional career (Kelly, 1978). Mentorship has been common in the business community for many decades, but the application of this concept to the health care field is fairly recent. Preceptorship differs somewhat from mentorship in that a shorter period of time is involved and the purpose of the relationship is rather specific.

Preceptorship has existed in nursing education since the 1960s (Mahr, 1979). It was first introduced in programs preparing primary health care practitioners. At that time physician preceptors were utilized for a clinical practicum involving extensive physical assessment skills. Today, many of the formal programs involving preceptorships are in elective baccalaureate level programs. The preceptor is generally a nurse from a speciality area, rather than a physician, and the focus is on skills in nursing process and interpersonal relations as well as those of physical assessment.

The use of preceptors in staff development is still relatively new. First mentioned in the literature as a method to orient new employees, this approach has spread throughout the full scope of staff development activities.

3

Just what is a preceptor? The word has been used to connote a number of different roles and functions—mentor, role model, master in the master-apprentice system. In reality, the preceptor functions to some extent in all of these, but the term has come to mean (in staff development circles) a particular person in a specific role. The preceptor is a person, generally a staff nurse, who teaches, counsels, inspires, role models, and supports the growth and development of an individual (the novice) for a fixed and limited amount of time with the specific purpose of socialization into a new role. The careful pairing of a novice with an experienced, precisely chosen staff nurse in the clinical setting provides an environment of nourishment and growth for the novice and of recognition and reward for the preceptor.

PRECEPTORSHIP TODAY

A variety of factors have evoked the recent interest in the preceptorship concept. These include changes in the economic environment, the relative inability of new nurse graduates to assume full patient care responsibilities, and the lack of opportunities for experienced nurses for advancement on a clinical level.

Today's economic environment is becoming more and more restrictive. No longer can we afford to spend vast sums on dubious efforts. Changing consumer attitudes and federal reimbursement reforms make control of resources and expenses of paramount importance. Failure to contain costs will result in economic suicide for any health care facility.

To add to this economic problem, new graduates are often unable to assume full patient care responsibilities. While their background may have a strong theoretical base, they lack experience and expertise in putting theoretical concepts to work. Educated for the ideal situation, new graduates often find themselves overwhelmed with the responsibilities and limitations of the real world.

More and more is expected of today's professional nurses. In addition to being experts in their area of practice, they are expected to be highly trained technicians, expert in the handling of a multiplicity of sophisticated monitoring and life support devices now common in hospitals. They are expected to be able to make split-second life-and-death decisions calmly and correctly, day after day. At the same time, nurses are to be warm, caring individuals concerned about each patient on a personal level. They must be skilled in communication, time management, and interpersonal relations. In addition, nurses must be cost conscious at all times—delivering high quality care for the least possible dollar amount. Finally, they must be willing and capable of doing this, not for the two or three patients they had as students, but for the five or six (or more) they will have as a regular staff member. Small wonder that new nurses find themselves overwhelmed.

Experienced nurses also find themselves at a disadvantage. Advancement for the nurse who desires to remain at the bedside is still limited. Only recently has any advancement been possible except by moving from the bedside to teaching or administration. Opportunities for advancement on a clinical level are increasing, but the most prestigious and remunerative positions in nursing are still in administration and education. The recent efforts of the profession to upgrade professional status and pay and to examine methods of professional retainment and advancement reflect an increasing awareness of these needs and of their effect on the profession as a whole.

These factors have led to one inevitable conclusion. Nursing administrators and educators must find innovative and effective ways of developing and rewarding nursing talent and expertise or face demise of the profession. A broad range of ideas and arrangements has been explored to accomplish this end. And a surprising number of them, in one format or another, incorporate the idea of preceptorship. By utilizing one individual's talent and expertise to develop another's, preceptorship can provide solutions to a variety of common institutional and individual needs that stem from the circumstances we have noted. Before considering specific ways in which a preceptor program can benefit both individuals and institutions, let us examine the specific roles and functions of the preceptor more closely.

THE ROLE OF THE PRECEPTOR

What roles does the preceptor fulfill? While there may be many specific responsibilities depending on the setting in which preceptors function, there are four major areas of responsibility. These are clinical practice, teaching, consulting, and research (see Figure 1-1).

Clinical Practice

For the most part, an individual is selected as a preceptor on the basis of clinical skills as a practitioner. Personal clinical practice, for the preceptor as well as the novice, remains a concern throughout the relationship.

The primary function of any staff nurse is the planning and delivery of nursing care, and it is no different for the preceptor. Without clinical competence, the ability to effectively plan, deliver, and supervise patient care is in question. This does not mean that preceptors must be experts in all areas of practice. That is impossible given the complexity of health care today. It does, however, mean that they must be knowledgeable and clinically comfortable with the range of patients usually seen in the unit. They must have a thorough understanding of the underlying pathology, and must demonstrate an ability to care for the psy-

Figure 1-1 The Preceptor Model

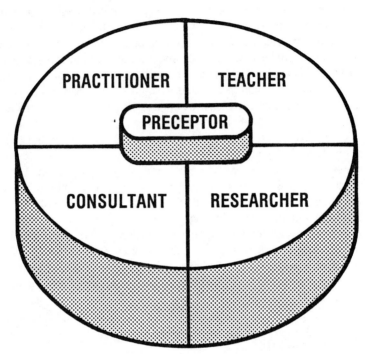

chosocial, cognitive, perceptual, cultural, and spiritual as well as biophysical needs of clients. Finally, since nursing practice rests on the application of the nursing process, the preceptor must demonstrate both understanding of and the ability to apply that process in both routine and complex nursing situations.

As a competent, skilled practitioner, the preceptor serves as a role model for the novice. New practitioners must have the opportunity to observe and critically examine requisite behaviors before trying them out. This can happen only if the clinically competent staff nurse is willing to be observed and questioned and has the capability of explaining detailed rationales and thought processes to the novice. This requires self-confidence and a willingness to examine one's own behavior. Both are crucial to the success of the preceptor's efforts.

Teaching

In addition to being a clinical practitioner, a preceptor is a teacher. Indeed, the primary difference between the normal staff nurse and the preceptor lies in the assumption of the teacher role. This includes identification of learning needs in conjunction with the learner, the planning and implementation of activities to meet those needs, and evaluation. Skillful staff nurses already display many of these behaviors in patient teaching and in interactions with new staff or students on the unit. They interpret as well as acquaint individuals with protocols, policies, and procedures, and assist learners to build the skills necessary for effective functioning on the unit. Patience and an open, inquiring attitude on the part of the preceptor are essential prerequisites. Specific skills such as needs identification or performance evaluation can be learned by a willing preceptor.

Consultation

Consulting is a role that is present throughout the preceptor's professional life. Most individuals have served as a resource for colleagues and friends before becoming preceptors. In the precepting relationship, initially, the preceptor serves primarily as a role model and teacher. Then, as the novice gains self-confidence, the role of teacher diminishes and that of resource person replaces it. Ultimately, teaching is superseded almost entirely by consulting and the novice joins other staff in their use of the nursing expert as a resource. For this to happen the person selected as a preceptor must be willing to "let go" of the novice, and to support and encourage independent growth. This is the kind of person who makes the preceptor system truly successful.

Research

The final function of the preceptor is research, although not in the traditional formal scientific manner. The established staff nurse is constantly involved in informal research. Which method works best for this patient? Have I tried that technique? The perpetual search for effective nursing interventions based on scientific principles and past experience embodies the spirit if not the letter of research methodology. The investigation of the novice's learning needs and the search for methods or experiences with which to meet those needs are other examples of the preceptor's research.

INTEGRATION INTO CURRENT NURSING SYSTEMS

The assumption of these roles by skilled staff nurses can benefit both institutions and individuals. However, unless adaptable to a broad range of requirements, preceptor systems could be severely limited. Fortunately, such systems fit into a broad range of situations and settings. Size of institution, method of care delivery, and specific need influence methods of implementation and utilization but do not affect the viability of preceptor programs.

Setting

Preceptor systems are in operation in a wide variety of settings. The utilization of preceptors in the preparation of primary health care practitioners continues today. Moraldo (1977) refers to some 70 preceptorship programs available for preparation of such practitioners in a variety of fields. References to preceptor programs for staff development are far scarcer but sufficient examples exist to allow general categorizations.

All sizes and types of facilities have been involved in preceptorship—from large, urban teaching institutions to small community hospitals. In addition, all types of practice have been included: medical-surgical, obstetrics, pediatrics, critical care and operating room, to name a few. As these examples come from the little that has been published in the field, one can only imagine the additional ways that are being developed but that have not yet been described in the literature.

Care Delivery System

Preceptors fit well into a variety of health care delivery system models. They may be used with equal success in functional, team, modular, total patient care, and primary nursing care structures.

Functional nursing, stemming from the work efficiency studies of the 20s, 30s, and 40s (Fairbanks, 1980), has today largely been replaced by other models but variations still exist in the practice world. Functional nursing organizes nursing care by job task, using, for example, a medication nurse, a treatment nurse, and a baths nurse. A preceptor, guiding the neophyte, can quickly and efficiently introduce the preferred method of doing the task and can role model organization so that all treatments, baths, etc. are attended to.

Team nursing was introduced following World War II. Growing out of behavioral management theories, the team approach promised a more effective method of care delivery and its use spread rapidly throughout the nursing community. The team consists of one professional nurse (the team leader) who helps other team members (RNs, LPNs, aides) provide care for a group of patients and assigns patient care according to patient need and staff ability. Ideally, this approach utilizes staff members to their full potential and promotes team member growth. A weak or disorganized team leader, however, can throw the system into disarray.

While allowing integration of the new team leader, a preceptor program provides a check and balance system to the ultimate benefit of the patient. It validates the authority of the new team leader through the acceptance and endorsement coming from a nurse familiar to all on the unit, promoting more rapid integration into the staff than might otherwise occur while still providing a means for monitoring and revising performance. This approach reduces or eliminates behaviors such as ignoring the new team leader in favor of someone known—"someone I know I can trust and who I know will do something about my problem." In addition, the use of one preceptor allows the novice to progress from team member to team leader while still relating to and following the role model of one individual.

Modular nursing is an offshoot of team nursing and employs a similar philosophy in a scaled-down version—two or three nurses providing care for a smaller group of patients arranged either geographically or by disease category (pulmonary patients, for example). Patient need and staff ability determine whether the module leader concentrates primarily on supervisory activities or on direct patient care.

Total patient care and primary nursing both utilize one nurse to plan and care for a group of patients. The difference between the two lies in the time frame. Total patient care implies responsibility and accountability for eight hours; primary nursing for twenty-four hours, with care delegated to associates when the primary nurse is not physically present. Preceptors fit ideally into this system. By taking a regular or slightly adjusted caseload, shared by novice and preceptor, the novice has the opportunity to observe and then practice the complex skills required for holistic practice. As the novice progresses, the preceptor can devote more time to assisting the novice with specific skills, the ultimate goal being that the novice assumes the entire caseload. This slow, gradual building eliminates stress on the novice while allowing progression as rapidly as possible. As the preceptor already knows and has an established rapport with the patients, attention can be focused primarily on the learner. In addition, the preceptor can intensively role model interpersonal and communication skills.

Preceptorship may indeed be a valuable extension of the staff development department. By introducing the new staff member in an organized manner under the direction and supervision of one individual, the opportunity exists to "try out" different behaviors in order to discover those that work best within the particular framework. At the same time, individual preceptors have a vested interest in seeing "their" novice succeed and share knowledge and information to that end. This does not always occur when a new person joins the staff. Knowledge about who to call for what and how to manipulate the system often becomes as important as technical know-how, yet it is just this information that is generally lacking in orientation programs. When one individual (the preceptor) works with the novice for a length of time, such knowledge is communicated and is not neglected because "everyone knows that" or through a lack of continuity.

Many institutions today have adopted the concept of a clinical ladder. This system of multiple layers of varying clinical skill levels recognizes expert clinicians and provides a means for clinical advancement. In addition to title and status advances, some form of economic remuneration is common.

Preceptorship fits extremely well into a clinical ladder model. It need not be added as a separate element or additional structure but can be incorporated as an integral responsibility in one or more of the advanced levels. This approach utilizes all the talents and expertise of the expert practitioner, provides rewards for the acquisition of that expertise while allowing the practitioner to remain at the bedside, and provides a methodology to share knowledge with novices in an efficient and effective manner.

THE BENEFITS OF PRECEPTORSHIP

To the Institution

A preceptor program attracts professional staff. Recruitment of qualified staff is essential to the quality and quantity of care provided by the institution, yet for many institutions it is a major difficulty. With a well-defined preceptor program, the institution has a drawing card that says to the prospective employee "We're interested in and care about you."

Even more vital than recruitment is the retention of current employees. Given the present economic climate and cost of orienting each new nursing employee, no institution can afford to lose its current staff. Opportunities for advancement, increasing responsibilities, and a supportive environment are essential to retaining qualified staff. A preceptor program provides a forum for these requirements. It recognizes and rewards the individual for achievement, provides a challenging environment for learning and growth, gives the preceptor added responsibilities and promotes advanced practice while allowing practitioners to remain at the bedside. Providing a professional environment that allows individual recognition without removing the nurse from the bedside has proved to be an effective method of retaining qualified staff.

Furthermore, preceptor programs provide motivation for all nursing staff. The constant reappraisal of practice and review of scientific rationale for that practice is beneficial for all professionals. The atmosphere of constant learning that is generated by the novices' presence stimulates learning on everyone's part. The enthusiasm and commitment exhibited by the preceptors are infectious, and spread to other staff. The result is enhanced morale, increased motivation for learning, and improved quality of care.

To Staff Development

Quality care and its support are expensive. Staff development departments, like many other hospital departments these days, are overcommitted and under-funded. The rising costs of health care and constant pressures for cost containment are impacting all health care institutions. Recent articles point to the role of nursing in general, and staff development in particular, in cost containment (Sovie, 1980).

Given this environment of cost awareness in an era of increasing specialization and skyrocketing technology, it becomes more and more difficult to provide a formal orientation program that meets the needs of all within a reasonable time frame. When one considers that it costs upwards of $5,000 to orient one new nursing employee (Sovie, 1980), and even more to orient personnel to critical care areas, the discovery of methods to reduce costs becomes crucial. Utilizing preceptors can decrease amounts of time spent in orientation periods for both experienced and new graduate nurses and can put to best advantage time spent on unit orientation, capitalizing on new employees' strengths and planning to meet their identified needs.

Preceptorship allows a decentralized form of orientation, permitting an ab-breviated formal orientation program. Such a program can cover only those areas of information needed by all participants and provide a formal mechanism for the specialized orientation and knowledge needed by practitioners in vastly dif-ferent types of clinical units. At the same time, a built-in method for validation of clinical skills is provided—an ever-present consideration for nursing educators in this litigation-conscious era.

Staff development personnel frequently make crucial decisions regarding an individual's clinical performance. Those decisions are often based on scant ob-servations. It is impossible for any staff development person to personally su-pervise every minute of an individual's orientation. Rarely is written documentation on performance available except in incident reports. Rare also is information on the type and amount of counseling, if any, given to the novice unless initiated by staff development instructors—an awkward task when done in retrospect and without seeing the behaviors involved. As a result, instructors often feel they are making decisions based on insufficient data, even if the novice's performance is conscientiously discussed with everyone involved.

Use of a preceptor eliminates many of these problems. Preceptors become very knowledgeable about their novices' performance. Working closely with the individual novice, they see the full range of behaviors utilized by the novice in a variety of situations. Intensity and length of observation combine to make the preceptor the best evaluator of the novice's progress. Counseling, if necessary, can be done at the time the problem arises by the individual who observed it— the preceptor. This observer is in a much better position to know all the facts and circumstances surrounding an incident than is the nurse educator, who "just popped up for a minute or two to see how things are going." Furthermore, the preceptor is in the best position to know all the strengths as well as weaknesses of the novice, and to be able to put particular incidents into context.

A system such as this makes effective use of all involved. It allows the staff development department to extend its services to a broader population, thus meeting a greater variety of institutional needs. By allowing a decentralized orientation, it provides a forum for the development of the specialized knowledge needed in today's hospitals. Efforts of staff development instructors may be directed at the problems or needs of the individual that truly require their expertise rather than trying to meet everyone's needs and meeting none of them effectively. Finally, it provides a mechanism for thorough follow-up and assessment of each new employee, an area often neglected.

To the Head Nurse

Head nurses also find a variety of benefits in a preceptor program. First, such a program allows them to upgrade and recognize their outstanding staff members without significantly impacting their budget. It provides a job enrichment program for those staff members, aiding in retention and the prevention of burnout. Second, it provides a formal, structured program to assist in orientation of new staff members, facilitates their social integration into the unit, and speeds their transition into fully functioning members of the unit. A preceptor also frees head nurses from some of the responsibilities of orientation, allowing them to concentrate on significant points or skills they wish to validate personally. At the same time, head nurses are assured that routine material is being taught in a systematic manner and that one person is responsible and accountable for getting this done. The head nurse is provided with an opportunity to observe the behaviors, skills, and learning ability of new staff members and to receive detailed validation of those behaviors, skills, and abilities from the preceptor.

Third, the head nurse benefits from the motivation and interest generated by the preceptor system. The atmosphere of learning and growth has a positive impact on all staff within the unit. Fourth, the preceptor supplies the unit with an individual having both clinical and educational ability. Judicious use of that resource enables head nurses to motivate and develop all members of their staff.

To the Preceptee

Benefits also exist for the individual being precepted. A comprehensive orientation program, geared to individual needs, can be planned. The novice is able to gradually learn the routines and practices of the institution without pressure for immediate assumption of a full patient load. This approach reduces stress, thus enhancing learning.

Through use of a preceptor, continuity of educational approach is achieved. One person provides an immediate resource for questions and clarification of information, and a minimum of time need be spent on material already familiar. A role model for the skills and behaviors best suited to the institution is provided, and individual attention can be given to the novice. In addition, a preceptor provides an instant friend, and an entree to the social system that exists on the unit and in the institution.

In addition to anxieties about being accepted as staff members, novices frequently have difficulty dealing with today's more involved and knowledgeable consumer. Today's nurses must be willing to answer questions and to actively involve patients in decisions regarding their care. The preceptor, working intensively with an individual novice, can assist that novice in polishing the full range of cognitive, psychomotor, and affective behaviors required for effective functioning as an established staff nurse.

To the Preceptor

Numerous benefits exist for the preceptor. Preceptors gain recognition and visibility from both peers and supervisors for their expertise, yet they are able to remain at the bedside if they so desire, or gain the visibility needed before moving toward management or educational positions. Either may prove invaluable in the advancement of the preceptor's career.

Many preceptors feel an inner satisfaction when watching the growth and development they have stimulated in the nurses they have worked with. The feeling of watching a previously hesitant novice skillfully manage a caseload of difficult patients is one that can't be expressed in words.

Another advantage for preceptors is the environment created by having a novice. Opportunity exists for growth on the part of both participants. Many preceptors enjoy the atmosphere of questioning and learning that surrounds the relationship, saying that it helps them to keep from feeling stale or stagnant.

Finally, the relationship between preceptor and novice can be an extremely satisfying one and may last as friendship long after the preceptor-preceptee association has ended. This stimulates development of a peer network that may provide advantages and benefits long after both the novice and preceptor have terminated employment at the facility.

PRECEPTORSHIP IN ACTION

Orientation

A major use of preceptors today is for orientation of the new graduate nurse, often in an extended orientation (residency, internship) format. These programs vary widely in length and format but have one central theme. As we have noted, recent graduates, particularly those from associate degree or baccalaurate programs, have strong theoretical backgrounds but lack experience in putting those concepts to work. In addition, new graduates normally have limited skills in technical procedures, leadership, and organization of care for groups of patients. These factors combine to make the transition from student to staff nurse a difficult one. The problem has become a focus of interest in the last decade, and has been amply documented in such works as Kramer's *Reality Shock* (1974).

The extended orientation period is an attempt to deal with such difficulties. It provides time to practice clinical skills and at the same time allows the institution to guide new practitioners into biculturalism, facilitating adaptation of their philosophy and practice of nursing with the needs and expectations of the institution. The preceptor is a crucial link in this process, providing a role model of bicultural behavior while subtly guiding the novice into professional behavior patterns suited to both nurse and institution. Promotion of a nursing self-concept that integrates both educational and work values is essential to the mental well-being of the novice.

Preceptorship has also proved itself in the orientation of experienced nurses. This approach permits the institution to focus on the identified needs of new employees, allowing best use of previously acquired expertise while providing a mechanism for the validation of skills and a readily available resource to meet identified needs. Furthermore, the experienced nurse functions in a regular patient care area during this time and quickly becomes an accepted and productive member of the staff.

Continuing Education

Another use of preceptors in staff development is for the preparation of practitioners in speciality areas. Schools of nursing rarely prepare practitioners to function immediately in areas such as intensive care units, emergency departments, or operating rooms. Institutions also have found that one or more years of general medical or surgical background better prepare individuals to handle the complex skills and stresses associated with such a practice area (Moyer & Mann, 1979). As a result, interest in the use of preceptors as a cost-effective method of preparing such practitioners is growing. References to such programs in the literature are rare, but the number of unpublished programs described informally and discussed at workshops and conferences is growing.

An additional use of preceptors is for staff development. This may be formal or informal. Casual, one-to-one learning situations occur daily in health care institutions. No longer can nurses consider themselves as having finished learning when they finish school. Education in our modern, technological environment is a continuous and lifelong process. Preceptors, as recognized clinical and educational experts on their units, are frequently called on in informal teaching situations by both peers and supervisors. Their expertise and teaching skills provide quick, easy-to-understand explanations of procedures or patient care concerns. In many instances, this incidental teaching is a major component of the preceptor's role.

Finally, preceptors may be called on to work formally with certain employees—for example, the individual having problems in a specific area. The person who needs intensive one-to-one work to improve charting or assessment skills is an ideal candidate for a preceptor relationship. The continuity and guided experiences selected by the preceptor can often bring the employee to the required standard of performance quickly. With firm guidelines and only one person to account to, the employee's performance improves dramatically. The preceptor, rather than being a disinterested bystander to problems, has a vested interest in helping the individual succeed. This prevents the buck from being passed from person to person in the hope that "if we just wait long enough, they'll get rid of her."

Exhibit 1-1 lists some of the common responsibilities with which preceptors have been involved.

Exhibit 1-1 Common Responsibilities of a Preceptor

- Interprets and applies philosophy and objectives of nursing in relationships with personnel, patients, and families.
- Is familiar with content provided in orientation, residency, or remedial program; refers novice to material that is not familiar.
- Selects or assists novice and/or head nurse in selecting patient assignments; assists in planning care for those patients.
- Acts as co-caregiver or resource person with novice, encouraging independence as novice is ready. Acts as professional role model.

- Conducts nursing rounds to discuss nursing care requirements and plans for patients.
- Demonstrates and/or supervises nursing procedures or skills that are new to the novice.
- Observes and assists the novice to prepare and administer medications according to hospital guidelines.
- Explains procedures for preparing patients for diagnostic tests and X-rays. Refers novice to departmental manuals. Arranges for novice to accompany patient whenever possible.
- Discusses dietary policies and procedures. Refers novice to departmental manual and resource people.
- Demonstrates or supervises novice in placement, maintenance, and discontinuation of intravenous therapy.
- Utilizes resources within the institution and plans with the novice to meet learning needs of the patient.

Exhibit 1-1 continued

- Observes novice's performance, and participates in evaluation.

- Provides feedback to novice regarding positive and negative aspects of novice's perform-ance; identifies with novice ways to improve performance.
- Shares evaluation of observed performance with novice, staff education department, and head nurse when indicated.
- Recommends experiences that will assist the novice to develop skills and knowledges required.

SUMMARY

The use of preceptors as a resource in both clinical content and educational practice fulfills a variety of individual, departmental, and institutional needs. Such a system fits well into a variety of health care delivery systems and provides solutions to a multitude of problems commonly faced in health care today. In the next chapters, we will examine both the development of a preceptor program and the task of selecting and preparing a corps of preceptors.

REFERENCES

Fairbanks, J. (1980). Primary nursing: What's so exciting about it? *Nursing, 10*(11), 55–57.

Kelly, L.Y. (1978). Power guide—The mentor relationship. *Nursing Outlook, 26*(5), 339.

Kramer, M. (1974). *Reality shock: Why nurses leave nursing.* St. Louis: Mosby.

Mahr, D.R. (1979). RN preceptors: Do they help students in the OR? *AORN, 30*(4), 724–730.

Moraldo, P.J. (1977). Better nursing care through preceptorships. *RN, 40*(3), 69–71.

Moyer, G., & Mann, J.K. (1979). A preceptor program of orientation within the critical care area. *Heart & Lung, 8*(3), 530–534.

Sovie, M. (1980). The role of staff development in hospital cost control. *Nurse Educator, 5*(6), 25–28.

Determining Need and Appropriateness

In Chapter 1 the concept of preceptors was examined and some of the various applications for preceptors described. In this chapter we will look at the questions you need to ask in order to decide whether you really want a preceptor program.

Preceptor programs are not for everyone and everything. They are not a panacea for all administrative or educational woes and they will not solve all problems. They may, in fact, create new difficulties. Preceptor programs fit a variety of applications admirably and can eliminate many of the common stumbling blocks faced by today's hospital administrators. However, preceptors are not the sole solution and their potential benefits must be weighed against the time, personnel, and monetary outlay required.

How, then, does one decide if such a program is what is needed? Let us first examine when preceptor programs are pertinent and should be contemplated.

WHEN TO EMPLOY A PRECEPTOR PROGRAM

Preceptor programs are pertinent whenever there are significant numbers of persons to be socialized into the same new role over a period of time. Preceptors have been utilized successfully for new graduate nurses, management personnel, operating room staff, new employees, new critical care staff, nurse practitioners, and the like. Consider implementing a preceptor program whenever it is necessary to repeatedly introduce individuals to the same role.

This is not to imply that only groups of learners are suitable for preceptor programs. Selection and development of an individual employee may be desired, as is often the case with management personnel, where it may be unusual to have more than one new manager at a time. A preceptor program can be ideal for this situation, providing a support system while promoting the best use of previously acquired skills. The key lies in using the same preceptor or corps of preceptors over a period of time and in not planning a single-time use.

The same preceptors may serve for a variety of learners. In many organizations preceptors are vital to a number of programs and duties may overlap. For example, there may be programs utilizing preceptors for new graduate nurses, critical care nurses, orientees, and nurses returning to nursing after having been away for several years (refreshers). The same preceptor pool might serve the new graduates, refreshers, and experienced orientees, and a similar but smaller pool serve the new critical care staff and its residency program.

The underlying principle of preserving the one-to-one relationship between the individual preceptor and learner for as long as necessary and of not expecting the same preceptor to facilitate learning for more than one individual at a time must be retained. It can be appropriate to use the same preceptor for more than one type of learner, provided that expectations for the learners are clear and the roles are familiar ones for the preceptors.

WHEN NOT TO EMPLOY A PRECEPTOR PROGRAM

When are preceptor programs not pertinent? In general, whenever they will be one-time efforts or when the numbers of persons to be socialized would overwhelm the system.

A one-time use of preceptors is usually not practical. Developing preceptors is time consuming and therefore expensive. When it is possible to spread the expense out over a period of time, preceptors often become significantly less expensive *in the long run*. A singular use destroys this long-term potential and may prove to be an extremely expensive effort.

Moreover, there is the difficulty of using *only* novice preceptors. Like anyone else, preceptors improve with practice. Denying ongoing experience prevents preceptors from refining their skills. This means that greater amounts of time are required of the coordinator, potentially increasing cost. Furthermore, using preceptors a single time may jeopardize desired outcomes.

Ordinarily, once a preceptor program is up and running, there will be a preponderance of seasoned preceptors. This allows the coordinator to concentrate efforts on assisting new preceptors. Potential preceptors will have had the opportunity to watch other preceptors in action and will therefore be better prepared to begin precepting than the initial preceptors were. Usually, the difficulties and expense of a one-time use outweigh the benefits.

Preceptors are also impractical in situations where the potential number of learners exceeds that of preceptors. The preceptor-learner relationship should be a one-to-one association; don't be deluded into thinking it can easily be extended. Preceptors must be available for novices to observe and critically examine desired role behaviors and they must be readily accessible to answer questions, clarify rationales, and translate the thought processes behind their actions. Opportunities to investigate the novice's learning needs, explore experiences to meet those needs, teach, and evaluate must be provided. When preceptor responsibilities are added to an existing staff nurse load, even if lighter than usual, effectively facilitating for more than one learner at a time is difficult if not impossible.

Inevitably, exceptions exist to the general rules given above. Primarily, exceptions involve the single-use rules. If an individual can function as a preceptor without a significant amount of development, it is possible to use him or her for a single situation (e.g., a new management person or a problem employee). Again, the potential preceptor must clearly understand and convey expectations for the novice, be accustomed to the role the novice is to assume, and feel comfortable in teaching situations.

FEASIBILITY

By now, perhaps you've decided a preceptor program is pertinent to your organization's needs. How then, do you decide if such a program is feasible?

Preceptor programs require both resources and support. An examination of six factors—leadership availability, administrative support, coordinator time, availability of preceptors, flexibility, and economics—can help you determine if a preceptor program is feasible for your facility.

Leadership

A committed, motivated leader is the first requirement. Unless at least one person is receptive to the concept of preceptorship and dedicated to making the program a success, the project is doomed to an early death. This is the individual who pulls the program together, fights for it, and makes it work. He or she must be skilled in the management skills of planning, leading, organizing, controlling, and decision making and knowledgeable regarding interpersonal relations, organizational behaviors, budgeting, and communications. Most of all, the leader must be a person devoted to the development, implementation, and support of an ongoing program; someone who can pull divided sides together, interpret rationale, motives, and methodology and still retain perspective, sanity, and a sense of humor.

Support

The potential to obtain administrative support is essential. This is not to imply that automatic approval should be granted to any preceptor program. It does mean that there must be an open mind on the part of administration and a willingness to listen and give the project a fair hearing.

Administrators will need to be convinced of the merits of your plan. The ability to put together and present a convincing argument and strategy for the program is a requirement for the person spearheading the undertaking. There may well be debate, but this often clarifies ideas and defines them into a workable model. Knowing that the plan will be fairly listened to and that there will be a readiness to examine alternatives to traditional approaches is a definite plus. Strategies for gaining administrative support will be covered in Chapter 3.

Coordination

Someone must be available for program coordination. Commonly, this will be the leadership person identified as the first necessity. Particularly at the onset of the project, the two functions are likely to be combined, or the coordinator role is combined with other responsibilities. The roles are separated here because it is likely that division will be required at some point in the life of the program and the possibility needs to be considered and evaluated in the early stages of planning.

Preceptor programs require significant amounts of coordination time. All elements must be pulled together to work as a cohesive whole. The time requirement can become massive if numerous preceptors, learners, and managers are involved. One individual must be available to collaborate with all parties, to integrate schedules, and generally trouble-shoot. The absence of someone to fulfill this role will severely hinder the stability of the program.

The Preceptor Pool

No other element is as crucial as the availability of preceptors. Preceptors must be accessible both quantitatively and qualitatively if a program is to prosper.

What is meant by the quantitative availability of preceptors? Simply that there be sufficient preceptors to accomplish your goals. The relationship between preceptor and learner must be one-to-one for success; it cannot be extended. The nurturance role of a preceptor requires time, commitment, and large amounts of energy. To ask that this be spread among even two learners is unreasonable. Therefore there must be one preceptor available for each potential learner. Adequate numbers of preceptors are critical.

What is meant by qualitative availability? Solely that having preceptors does not mean having just the right number of warm bodies. Preceptors must be individuals who are appropriate role models. Novices will be socialized into the behaviors demonstrated by their preceptor. Before selecting each preceptor you must carefully consider whether this is a person whose behavior patterns you wish perpetuated. If the answer is no, then the individual is not a candidate for a preceptor role, regardless of how badly additional preceptors are needed. No other single step is as important as preceptor selection. It is infinitely more desirable to limit learners than to take too many and socialize them into undesirable behavior patterns. Eventually, as the learners mature in their role and themselves become sought as role models, the preceptor pool can expand. Hard as it may be, if there are insufficient role models for your needs, take fewer learners.

Flexibility

A major requirement for both the program administrator and coordinator is flexibility, the ability and willingness to adapt to change. Change is inevitable. The type of staff hired changes, necessitating changes in the format of your program. Preceptors come and go, requiring that new ones be identified and developed. As resources diminish and health care costs affect professional to nonprofessional staff ratios, patterns of care and expectations will change. Any of these may require revisions in the program's format or content. Each person involved in the program must be willing to openly examine the need for changes purposefully and deliberately.

Part of flexibility as it is discussed here is a willingness to be sensitive to the needs of the preceptors. Precepting is hard work; it requires constant amounts of energy, enthusiasm, and problem solving. Inevitably, preceptors will need breaks. It is unfair to everyone to use preceptors continually. It exhausts your preceptors, weakens your program, and jeopardizes the quality of instruction and support. Therefore, program coordinators must be alert to the subtle cues of fatigue and be flexible enough to program relief and/or variety into the scheduling.

Besides these, numerous other changes will be needed during the life of the program. If those involved in the program's management are not prepared to adjust to those changes, the program is condemned to failure.

Funding

Ultimately, we come to the fundamental issue of economics. Without sufficient financial support the program will wither and die. Sufficient monies for development, administrative and clerical staff, preceptor reimbursement (if desired), and learners' salaries must be available. Considerable attention will be devoted to budgeting for preceptor programs in Chapter 3.

Making the Decision

Several prerequisites for successful preceptor programs have been discussed. To decide for yourself whether a preceptor program is feasible for your setting, ask yourself the following questions:

1. Do I have more than one person to be oriented to the same role over a period of time? How many? How many roles?
2. Is a committed, motivated leadership person available or obtainable?
3. Is the administrative environment such that I could obtain support?
4. Is there someone available to serve as program coordinator?
5. Do I have personnel "on board" whom I would feel comfortable with as role models?
6. Are there sufficient role models to fulfill the program's needs?
7. Is our facility flexible enough to respond to changes within such a program as they become necessary?
8. Is the leadership person flexible enough to adapt to changes?
9. Is the potential coordinator flexible?
10. Is the economic environment such that financial backing for the project could be obtained?

SUMMARY

Preceptor programs are viable whenever there are numbers of persons to be socialized into new roles over a period of time. They require that resources such as leadership personnel, preceptors, administrative support, flexibility, and capital be available. The ten questions posed within this chapter helped you to decide whether a preceptor program is for you. The next chapter will look at the comprehensive planning required by the decision to pursue a preceptor program.

Chapter 3

Planning Your Program

The process of planning involves making many decisions. We could say you will have to determine the who, what, when, where, why, and how of your program.

There are three phases to planning: exploration, preparation, and introduction and education. Careful attention to each phase ensures comprehensive coverage of every detail and contributes to smooth and successful implementation. The first two phases, exploration and preparation, will be the focus of this chapter. Exhibit 3-1 provides an overview of the planning process.

EXPLORATION

The exploration phase began when you answered the questions posed in the last chapter. This phase also involves reviewing the literature, examining the prevailing organizational goals and philosophies, seeking administrative support, attending workshops and seminars, talking with people currently utilizing preceptor programs, and generally gathering information. Exploration ends with the drafting of a preliminary program plan.

Review the Literature

Reviewing the literature is a relatively simple task. While a comparatively large body of literature exists on the use of preceptors in formal education, publications on preceptor use in nursing staff development are limited in number. A variety of articles have been written that discuss the use of preceptors for specific staff development purposes. Reviewing these will help to stimulate ideas that may prove useful in the design of your program. (A selected bibliography can be found at the end of this book.)

Exhibit 3-1 The Planning Process

Exploration

- Review the literature
- Examine current organizational goals and philosophies
- Attend workshops and seminars
- Talk with people currently using preceptor programs
- Draft a preliminary program plan
- Secure preliminary approvals

Preparation

- Seek input from persons who will be involved or interacting with the program or its graduates.
- Develop a budget.
- Write performance descriptions.
- Determine evaluation methodologies.
- Revise program plan.
- Secure final approvals.
- Market your program (throughout the planning process).
- Select program personnel.
- Finalize a polished program plan.

Introduction and Education

- Select preceptor development approach.
- Select novices.
- Pilot the program.

Examine Organizational Goals

However useful the literature, the type of program you plan to institute must be congruent with organizational goals and philosophies. An examination of your goals and their relationship to organizational aims is crucial to determining the potential for administrative support. Review in detail your organization's goals and philosophies and define, either mentally or in writing, how your proposed program contributes to their accomplishment.

The key to obtaining administrative support is identifying why your program is needed. How is a preceptor program important to administration? Only by meeting the organization's particular needs or fostering its goals can you hope to obtain support. If the hospital is a profit-making one, for example, determine how your program can contribute to cost effectiveness or enhance the institution's reputation. If your program does not directly support institutional aims and objectives, you will have a much more difficult time obtaining support. Without this support, you cannot hope to succeed.

Seek Administrative Support

Obtaining administrative support is fundamentally an issue of marketing. Kotler (1972) defines marketing as "the set of human activities directed at facilitating and consummating exchange" (p. 12). This exchange need not include money. Goods, services, money, attention, energy, support, time, and information are all potential elements for exchange.

According to Kotler (1972), three conditions are necessary for successful marketing: (1) two or more parties must be potentially interested in making an exchange; (2) each party must possess something of interest to the other; and (3) each party must be capable of communication and delivery of the valued item.

Because the potential audience is so broad, we may break down marketing into two general areas—internal and external. Internal marketing refers to the selling of the program inside the facility or organization, external marketing to recruiting applicants and convincing those outside the facility of the value of the program. To be successful, both must be addressed. Internal marketing will be considered here, as it deals with obtaining administrative support, and external marketing will be discussed in the following chapter.

Internal marketing is crucial. From the conception of the program, marketing to the significant decision makers within the institution is essential if the program is to survive.

How do you market a preceptor program to those significant decision makers? While there is no one right answer for all situations, key principles can help you identify the "right" way for your setting.

First, consider all the ramifications of your program. When changes threaten the autonomy or security of others, there will be resistance. Attempt to anticipate where you will face resistance, and think out possible responses before they are needed. Answer objections in a cool, collected, and professional manner, openly acknowledging others' concerns. Discuss these concerns by responding rather than just reacting.

Maintain your own credibility. Be well informed about preceptor programs in general and your own program in particular. Be sure of your facts and get them straight. Lack of credibility damages your chances to obtain what you desire.

Establish an informal communication network. A timely and accurate information flow is essential. This means a flow not only downward but upward and across as well. Such a network will permit appropriate intervention when necessary and facilitate interchange among individuals, groups, and yourself.

Identify key people who are influential within the organization. Whose opinions are listened to and respected? Whose support is crucial to the program's success? An orientation program, for example, cannot succeed without the active support of the head nurses. The sooner those people can be apprised of your plans and incorporated into them where possible, the better your chances for success. Remember that people tend to support what they help to plan. Opinions and suggestions from this group can be invaluable during the planning phase, and identification of their concerns can help you anticipate and counteract those you will face from others. In addition, including these individuals gives them a vested interest in seeing the program obtain necessary resources and support. Once they are involved, even if only in an informal or advisory way, they are more likely to actively intervene on the program's behalf. Their support may mean the difference between implementing or abandoning your plans. (Once the preceptors are selected, don't forget that they are key people in the selling of your program. The more your preceptors know and can articulate about all aspects of the program, the better resource they'll be for persons who have questions or concerns.)

Be involved in the decision making that affects your program or know who is and lobby them. Above all others those individuals must understand the relevance of the program to organizational goals.

Be prepared to bargain or negotiate when necessary. It may be expedient to give up something in order to make an overall gain. For example, you really want four novices in a new graduate residency program but if it's a choice between two novices or none, or between two weeks of orientation or none, you'll settle for two. Decide beforehand where you are willing to bargain and where you will not compromise. Negotiating means compromise; by definition you'll be giving up something. Don't permit negotiations in areas where you aren't willing to compromise.

How can you convince others that your program is important? Basically, you must look at the program from their perspective. It's easy for you to see why you think the program is important but often these reasons have little relevance for people you need to convince. Why is the program important to them? Perhaps the program will recruit nurses for a director and an institution that is experiencing difficulties in recruiting nurses. Perhaps it will help to retain nurses who are leaving for more challenging positions elsewhere. Perhaps it is cost beneficial in terms of turnover and orientation expenses. What are the problems facing the individuals you are trying to convince and how will your program help them achieve their aims? Only by meeting their needs can you hope to convince others that the program is important to them. If the program will meet only your needs, it will have little chance for success.

When you meet resistance, be understanding. Find out what the person believes and why. Use active listening. Don't argue or contradict. Ask clarifying questions and be responsive rather than reactive. Often the concerns originally expressed are not truly the underlying worries. Explore for the "real" reasons and discuss them calmly and intelligently. Show others how they can benefit from your program and give them time to reflect. When they begin to express your ideas as their own, you'll know you've been successful.

Don't use jargon. If you are to be understood, you must speak the language of your listener. This may mean that you must familiarize yourself with their language (finance, for example) in order to be effective.

Be persistent. People don't change their thinking overnight. Repeated discussions may be necessary. You must be sure that you've been heard, and that the individual is seriously considering what you have said. If you lack credibility or influence with the individual, have someone he or she respects discuss the issue. This will often succeed where you might fail.

Survey the Field

Discuss preceptor programs with as many people as possible. Be outgoing. Search out opportunities to share what you are planning and doing and actively seek information from others. Attend workshops or seminars if they are available. Visit institutions that are using preceptors in ways similar to those you envision for your facility. This permits you to observe their systems in action and contributes testimony on their successes and failures. It also saves you both time and aggravation as you learn from others' mistakes.

Draft a Preliminary Program

Having done the above, you'll have a pretty good idea of whether your first ideas are workable, and will mentally have worked out an approach. The next step is to draft a preliminary program plan. Exhibit 3-2 provides a format for making notes on your plan.

The plan spells out in detail the who, what, where, when, why, and how of the program. It outlines in writing its purposes and objectives. Going through this procedure clarifies thinking and makes you get down to specifics.

Putting the plan in writing will undoubtedly raise questions in your mind. Make a note of these but don't let them delay the preparation of the first draft. After the plan is on paper for the first time, questions can be researched and needed or desired changes incorporated. There will always be unanswered or unanswerable questions. Don't let them delay your progress.

Some fundamental elements should be included in the program plan. These include:

Exhibit 3-2 Notes for Preliminary Program Plan

Purpose _____
_____

Applicants
  Who is the program designed for? _____
  Who may apply? _____
  Requirements? _____
  References? _____ Number _____ From Whom? _____
  Selection Process: Who selects _____
    Criteria? _____
    _____
    _____
    _____
    Process? _____
    _____

Program Length? _____ Frequency? _____
Program Location? _____
Preceptors: Qualifications and requirements _____
    _____
  Selection process: Who selects? _____
    Criteria? _____
    _____
    Process _____
    _____

Format? _____
_____

Responsibilities of Education: _____
_____
_____
_____

Responsibilities of Administration: _____
_____
_____
_____

Content Areas: _____
_____
_____

Objectives: _____
_____
_____
_____

Evaluation: _____
  Who is to be evaluated: _____
  By whom? _____
  Intervals _____
  Criteria _____
  _____

1. purpose of the program
2. program objectives
3. application requirements
4. employment conditions and benefits
5. program length and location
6. selection process for preceptors
7. evaluation procedures
8. the role of administration and education
9. content and format
10. specific objectives

You may also include why you are running the program and when you will do it. The reasons for running the program differ from the purpose in that the purpose defines exactly what you are trying to accomplish through the program; the reasons for running it delineate why the product is needed.

Purpose of the Program

The program's purpose derives from the circumstances that produced the need for the program. It should be presented in a short, comprehensive statement of the program's intent. For example: "To provide an extended clinical experience for the graduate nurse to prepare her for assuming the role of a registered nurse in an acute health care facility" (Selg & Morrow, 1981, p. 1). Or "To provide an organized system of cardiac education with curricula commensurate to each level of nurses' professional growth and development—from basic to advanced levels" (Ferris, 1980, p. 20).

This section should preface all other parts of the plan since anyone reading the plan will be interested first in what the program is trying to achieve.

Program objectives describe the specific goals of a particular program. Usually 2 to 6 in number, they outline in greater detail the program's purpose. For example: "To assist new nurses to develop leadership skills." "To make new nursing staff aware of hospital policies, procedures, and standards." "To acquaint professional nurses with the structure and organization of pre-hospital cardiac care."

Application Requirements

A definition of who will participate in the program should be included. It should outline not only who the program is designed for (e.g., new graduate nurses or new head nurses) but also who may apply or who is to be incorporated into the program (e.g., "any newly hired Memorial Hospital staff nurse" or "any graduate of an accredited school of nursing"). If applicable, the following should be included: (1) requirements for application (e.g., "one year medical or surgical experience in an acute care facility'' or ''possess or is eligible for current state licensure''); (2) what references will be needed, if any, and from whom (e.g., ''Two references will be required: one personal reference and one from the applicant's current manager or instructor''); (3) what the selection process will be (who selects, and on what criteria) (e.g., ''Applicants will be selected by the Director of Nursing Education on the basis of personal and professional references and personal interview''); and (4) the interviewing process (e.g., ''Individual interviews will be conducted during a two-week period one month before the start of the program''). Delineation of these elements will save time and target the program to those for whom it is intended.

Length and Location

The length and location of the program need to be defined. Where will the program will be carried out? Does it involve the entire hospital or only selected nursing units? Will novices rotate through units, giving them the opportunity to try out different clinical specialties and gain a variety of skills, or will they remain in one unit concentrating on developing one area of expertise? Also, what is the length of the proposed program? Early specification of the areas and the time required will help to clarify the scope of the project.

Although you will have an idea of how often you will want or need the program run, this will probably change periodically because of changing needs. If you include such information, your program plan will need to be rewritten each time you change your time frame. Therefore, it is sometimes preferable to be vague on this issue in the plan and save yourself the time and aggravation of frequent revisions.

Preceptors

The program plan also needs to discuss preceptors. It must describe the qualifications for preceptors and the process by which they will be selected. What are the requirements for someone who desires to become a preceptor? How will the selection be conducted, by whom, and using what criteria? Preceptor qualifications are covered extensively later in the chapter. For now, just jot down your preliminary thoughts regarding their selection.

Evaluation

The next area to be covered in your preliminary plan is evaluation. Will it be a formal or an informal process? By whom will evaluations be done, at what intervals, and using what criteria? Will only novices be evaluated or are preceptors to be rated also? You won't have given a great deal of thought to this aspect yet. Jot down your first thoughts. There will be opportunities to explore this aspect in depth later.

Organization: Roles and Design

The roles of education and administration must be outlined. Who will be responsible for which aspects of the program? Designating this early in the planning phase will allow everyone to examine expectations and, if there are conflicts, will permit alternatives to be found while there is still time to easily change the plan.

The organizational design will be a crucial element of the program. Several options are available: hiring of the novice and direct line authority through the unit's head nurse, hiring by nursing administration or education within a separate cost center and with line authority retained by them, or a variation of these. Each approach has unique advantages and disadvantages.

In many programs, whoever normally hires for the unit, the head nurse, for example, hires the novice. This is commonly the approach taken in orientation programs. Utilizing the established program for objectives and content, direct line authority over the novice is retained and their practice and progress are supervised. Normally, in such arrangements novices do not rotate to other areas or units, although they may rotate to other shifts.

Generally, this approach works well. It minimizes confusion over supervisory lines, allows new staff to become known by others on the unit, permits the manager to be more directly involved with the learner, and facilitates gaining of knowledge directly needed by novices for the areas where they will practice.

However, it is possible to lose the emphasis on the learner role, particularly if the unit is especially busy or short staffed. It is often difficult for managers to balance the dual roles of providing adequate care and supporting the learner. Unfortunately, at times the pressures of running the unit may cause the needs of the learners to become a secondary consideration, and thus the focus and benefits of the program may be lost.

An alternative approach is for nursing administration or education to hire the novices and support them out of a separate cost center until they are through the learning process. Although more complicated to organize, this arrangement has multiple advantages for programs such as internships or residencies.

First, retaining the novices in educationally or administratively controlled positions makes it more likely that control of the learning environment will be maintained. The focus is on learning rather than only providing care.

This raises another question. Will novices and preceptors be considered part of the normal staffing or will they be considered as extra personnel? As novices, it is difficult to carry a full load, and preceptors must have time to teach as well as take care of patients. However, it is extremely expensive to count neither in your staffing ratios. One solution is to count the preceptor and exclude the novice. This approach seems to reach a happy medium and has for the most part worked well in the clinical setting.

There are two further advantages to the centralization of novices. First, from a practical point of view, it is easier to control what is happening to and for the novices from one central location. Although interns or residents, for example, will undoubtedly be assigned to various units throughout the organization, having one "home base" facilitates making contact and communicating with them. Second, arranging for novices to operate out of a central pool gives head nurses the opportunity to observe their performance and style without having to hire them. This is appreciated, particularly if novices rotate through areas and head nurses can choose among several candidates. It also benefits the novices, as they have the opportunity to observe the different management styles of various head nurses in action and choose the approach they feel most comfortable with.

The greatest disadvantage to centralization is the visibility of cost. Many managers or administrators prefer to include the cost of orienting or training new staff, rather than to pull it out separately. If novices are hired into and paid through a separate cost center, this is impossible.

Content and Format

The next elements to be designated are the content areas to be included and the format for the program. Will the program involve clinical time only? Classes? What proportion of each? What are the content areas to be covered? Make your lists and be prepared to trim them down when priorities have been set.

Specific Objectives

Finally, identify specific objectives for the program. These objectives describe in behavioral terms what the novices should know or do at the end of the program. Objectives delineate the boundaries of subject matter and indicate how each area relates to the whole. Clear objectives remove ambiguity, allow learning activities to be chosen more precisely, and inform novices, preceptors, and managers about what is expected.

Well-written objectives include four elements: who will perform the behavior, the behavior desired, the level of acceptable behavior, and sometimes, conditions.

Who will perform the change in behavior is the first element of an objective. The subject of that change is the client for whom the program is intended, and objectives should start with identification of the person who will perform the change, i.e., "the novice," "the learner," "the participant," "the student."

A description of the behavior desired is next. This should consist of two parts: the actual behavior to be demonstrated and the result of the behavior. Action verbs should be used to describe the actual behavior, for example, to "list," "describe," or "demonstrate." The result of the behavior is a description of the actual task to be accomplished, for example, "list signs of congestive heart failure."

Taken together, these two elements describe what the learner should be able to do. For example, "The participant will be able to differentiate between grief and depression" or "The learner will be able to demonstrate correct body mechanics in giving patient care."

The level of acceptable behavior should be specified. The criterion, as it may be called, may include a time limit ("before the end of the program"), the amount of information to be covered ("four out of five questions"), or characteristics of performance ("according to hospital policy" or "using appropriate technique").

Finally, in some instances conditions may be included. The conditions describe relevant circumstances under which mastery of the task will be demonstrated, e.g., "given a case study," "after the class on body mechanics," or "on completion of the program."

When these elements are combined into one statement, a comprehensive description of what is expected is obtained; for example, "At the completion of the class on body mechanics, the participant will demonstrate correct body mechanics in giving patient care."

Domains. Objectives are classified according to the type of behavior called for. There are three areas of classification, called domains: cognitive, psychomotor, and affective. The domains provide a common frame of reference for looking at behavior and a framework for looking at the desired outcomes. Although separated, the domains are in reality never totally independent. They are classified on the basis of the dominant activity rather than on complete purity.

Cognitive objectives refer to thinking or knowledge. The largest number of educational objectives fall into this realm. To determine cognitive objectives, ask yourself "What does the learner need to know?"

Psychomotor objectives describe physical tasks or motor skills. To determine psychomotor objectives, ask yourself what activities the learner must be able to do.

Affective objectives describe what must be thought or felt. These are the most difficult objectives to formulate since they involve changes in attitude, and values and feelings are often internalized and difficult to measure. They also take the longest to achieve.

To see how each of these objectives fits together, let us look at the following example which has to do with nursing care plans.

1. Cognitive objective: "The learner will identify the four components of a nursing care plan according to hospital policy."
2. Psychomotor objective: "The learner will write at least two nursing care plans according to hospital policy during the second week of orientation."

3. Affective objective: "The participant will actively support the use of nursing care plans on the clinical unit."

It is easy to see how the domains overlap but how the dominant activity determines the domain.

Varying levels of complexity exist within the domains. The taxonomy of objectives given in Appendix D outlines these levels and provides examples and action verbs that will help you to write objectives for your program.

Levels. Program objectives may be written at three levels: overall program objectives, unit objectives, and instructional plan objectives.

Overall program objectives are goals that define the product of the program and give direction to all aspects of the program. They include the general objectives that direct teaching and preceptors in their activities.

Unit objectives describe smaller stages of development. For example, the overall program may cover ten weeks, and novices may change shifts or areas after four weeks and every two weeks after that. Unit objectives would describe what is to be accomplished in each of the divisions, i.e., during the first four weeks and each additional two weeks.

Instructional plan objectives describe even smaller levels of accomplishment. These might be objectives for particular classes or experiences, such as a day with IV therapy, or the preceptor's objectives for a particular day or period of time.

The amount of detail in the objectives depends on the type of novice you will have. The more mature and independent the novice, the less structure needs to be provided. For example, with new graduate nurses it may be desirable to outline objectives on a week-by-week basis, while with new managers, biweekly or even monthly time frames may be sufficient. Orientation programs sometimes omit unit level objectives altogether when the overall program objectives and those of the instructional plan are thought to offer sufficient structure. Use your judgment in deciding how detailed to be, remembering that too much structure is usually preferable to not enough.

Secure Preliminary Approvals

Now is the time to secure the preliminary approvals needed to continue further with the project. Normally, each institution or facility has an established procedure for securing approvals before beginning a new project or changing an existing one. Proceed through the steps as outlined for your facility or institution.

PREPARATION OF THE PROGRAM

When preliminary approvals are granted, you'll be ready to move on to the second phase of planning—preparation. This is the phase of gathering input from people who will be involved with the program, developing a preliminary budget, writing performance descriptions if applicable, completing a polished program plan, and securing final approvals.

Seek Input

The first step of preparation is to seek input from a variety of people who will be directly involved with the program. Discuss with them its goals, objectives, content, and format. What do they think the program should accomplish? How long do they think it will take? Should the program consist of classes or will a purely clinical focus better meet the needs of those concerned? You already have an idea of what you want the program to encompass and can explore your ideas and discuss theirs in light of your preliminary design. This helps to clarify and solidify thoughts and approaches.

Try to include those individuals who will be influential in making the program a success and those who will be working with its graduates. Their early involvement in the planning will help focus the program to meet their perceived needs and will ultimately contribute to its success. Individual interviews, group interviews, or a brainstorming session are all possibilities. The best way to gather input will be based on the individuals involved.

Design a Budget

A major part of the preparation is design of a budget. Your case will be considerably strengthened if you do your homework well. Even in a preliminary budget you will need to estimate expenses and project revenue needed to support the program.

There are two purposes for budgeting: coordination and cost control. Coordination of the program's budget with those already in existence helps to avoid duplication and contributes to efficient use of services and resources. Cost control is of vital interest to all health care organizations today, given the current economic climate. Administrators are concerned with delivering high quality services for the lowest possible dollar amount. A carefully developed budget assists you in gathering support for your project and reflects favorably on your ability to plan and manage a program.

Evaluating Budgetary Needs

A number of factors need to be considered when evaluating your budgetary needs. These include the type of patient population the institution serves, personnel policies, nursing care standards and procedures, and the program's goals and objectives.

Patient conditions, volume, age groups, and care expectations potentially affect your program and thus influence its monetary needs. With the majority of reimbursement arrangements dependent in part on patient volumes, numbers of patients served within the institution have direct correlations with the amounts and proportions of monies available. The nature of the institution's clientele dictates the types of novices you can prepare. What diagnoses and age groups do your patients encompass? Are they primarily inpatients or outpatients? What are your average length of stay and acuity? These determine the type of program you can support, since they dictate the resources available to run the program and the numbers and expertise of staff necessary to support it.

Organizationally determined factors also have implications for your program. Policies and procedures, staff ratios, and methods of care delivery influence the program's design and operation and thus its financial needs.

Personnel policies have obvious implications for budgeting. What are current policies on salaries, overtime, normal work hours (and the flexibility of those hours), and education time? Are those policies likely to change in the next six months or year? Do they affect your program? What financial resources will be needed?

Nursing care standards and procedures are also factors. What are the standards of care within the institution? Are they uniform throughout all the nursing areas? Do managers, education personnel, and staff operate from the same value system? What are the formal and informal sanctions imposed for violation of those standards? Standards of care are based on the prevailing value system. Conflicts of values between management, educators, preceptors, or novices will pose multiple problems for the program and will require additional resources.

What is the primary method of patient assignment? This has particular impact if one is preparing graduate nurses. Most of today's new nurses are educated with the preponderance of their experience in either total patient care or primary nursing systems. Therefore, if your institution uses primarily team nursing, or expects persons to revert to it when necessary, it will take longer for novices to become proficient than if you are using only the other two modalities. The implications for budgeting are obvious.

Staffing patterns are also to be considered. RN ratios, educational and experiential levels, management expectations of staff, and vice versa all play a part. The number of skilled personnel available in your community and in the institution will dictate, in part, the need for your program. Education affects value systems, and experience affects productivity. More acutely ill and complex patients require more skilled nursing hours and demand more from novices. In addition, equipment availability and the presence or absence of support systems for non-nursing tasks affect the availability of nursing personnel for patient care and guidance of novices.

Two other factors must be considered. First, what are the goals and philosophies of your program? What do you hope to accomplish? Beginning-level proficiency, for example, will demand a different level of resources than advanced competency. Your budget must reflect your goals.

Second, what is the preparation level of those entering your program? It will take less time to orient experienced staff nurses to your institution, for example, than to orient a new graduate to assume full patient care responsibilities.

All of these factors are significant in budgeting since they influence the nature and availability of staff and the type of program that can be supported. The impact of each must be considered when projecting your budgetary needs. Exhibit 3-3 will help you summarize these factors for your program.

Getting Down to Work

Before beginning the budget, it is crucial to decide whether the program will be added to an existing department (the most likely option) or whether a new department will be created. This has a substantial impact on budget planning. Since adding a preceptor program to an existing department often has minimal

Exhibit 3-3 Factors To Consider in Budgeting

FACTOR	DESCRIPTION	IMPACT
Patient population		
Personnel policies		
Patient care delivery system		
Nursing standards and procedures		
Goals and objectives of program		
Other		

financial impact, we will concentrate on the more comprehensive new department approach, although it is less likely to be used.

Budgets are normally discussed and planned on a yearly basis but there is no absolute requirement to do so. If budgeting is new to you, it may prove easier to plan on a three- to six-month basis and then evaluate your progress. Discuss possible options with the facility's financial officer or other person responsible for budget planning.

Preparation

First, become acquainted with the planning process and budgeting forms used at your facility, if you are not comfortable with them already. While the format is usually slightly different at each institution, budgets generally contain three main sections: personnel, or manpower, needs (normally the largest proportion); operations, which support ongoing needs for supplies and equipment; and capital expenses, or major monetary outlays. Most institutions have a cutoff point—say at $100.00, above which operating expenses become capital expenditures. You will need to know which section of the budget should be used. For example, if you are buying six videotapes at $75.00 each, are they to be considered as one capital expense or six operational expenses?

The next step is to examine past budgets of programs such as you propose (if any exist). This analysis can help you identify equipment that has previously been purchased and pinpoint areas for change. Were the monies set aside sufficient? Did they meet the needs of the program adequately? What type of items were included? Such knowledge will be helpful in drawing up your budget.

More often than not, previous budgets do not exist and you must start from scratch. If you are on your own when it comes to proposing a budget for your program, where do you begin?

Manpower Costs

Start by estimating staff needs. Manpower will probably be the largest cost within your budget. Who are your personnel? How many hours will they be working for the program? At what cost per hour? Will you need additional personnel? Consider administrative and coordinator positions as well as preceptors and novices. If staff to run the program will be pulled from existing personnel, must they be replaced? Recruiting one of your best staff nurses to coordinate may be a great idea until you realize that it leaves you without a preceptor on that unit. Will secretarial assistance be needed? Consider wages for classes and meetings as well as clinical time and remember to include the hidden costs that fit into this category.

Benefits are a substantial "hidden" cost in any personnel budget. Most institutions have a standard percentage that they use to calculate the cost of benefits—for example 25 percent on top of the hourly wage. Sick time, overtime, and replacement time must also be provided for. Replacement time is that time (money) used to replace persons when they are ill, on leave, or on vacation. Salary rates or ranges can normally be obtained from the personnel department, or the general rate of pay that prevails within the area can be solicited by calling other facilities. Use these as the guidelines for calculating salaries and wages.

Some salaries and wages may be negotiable, depending on the type of novice you are considering. In many instances, standard wage scales or union contracts will apply. In some situations, however, it may be possible to establish a special pay grade for the novices. For example, several of the hospitals in the Seattle area have a graduate nurse resident pay scale lower than that for the first grade of registered nurses. Explore what is common in your area before you finalize your wages.

As each category of staff must be examined independently, next consider the preceptors. Should they receive extra pay? There are two schools of thought. One holds that precepting is part of the normal job description of the professional nurse and therefore no special remuneration should be provided. The other holds that precepting is "above and beyond" normal responsibilities and that therefore special compensation is deserved—more responsibility deserves more pay. Some institutions have incorporated precepting into their clinical ladder; it is part of the normal responsibility for the level of performance and the higher level of performance is rewarded commensurately. Others pay for some levels of precepting, for example, residents or interns, but not for others, such as experienced staff nurses orienting to the unit. The preferred approach depends on the philosophy and financial resources of each institution, and must therefore be settled individually by each facility.

Similar principles apply to instructors and program administration staff. Ascertain the common salary range or hourly wage for the positions included and budget accordingly. The first part of the budget projection sheet (Exhibit 3-4) will help you project the manpower costs of your program.

A further aspect of manpower cost, estimation of development cost, is the next step in the budgetary process. This is the cost of actually developing materials and content for the program. In reality, it also includes the cost of preparing your program plan and budget. In addition, it covers the expenses of interviewing program personnel, recruiting, interviewing and selecting novices, selecting and training preceptors, and the development of materials, such as evaluation forms, needed within the program.

To estimate development cost, make a comprehensive list of the materials your program will need. Include such items as preparing job descriptions, evaluation forms, and the program plan. Then estimate the number of hours it will take to develop those materials. Be generous—remember it always takes at least one and a half times as much time as you think it will. Be sure to allow time

Exhibit 3-4 Estimating Program Budget

PERSONNEL COST	Estimated Hours	Bene-fits	Other	Cost/ Hour	Estimated Cost
Administrative person					
Development	___	___	___	___	___
Ongoing	___	___	___	___	___
Program coordinator					
Development	___	___	___	___	___
Ongoing	___	___	___	___	___
Preceptors					
Training	___	___	___	___	___
Ongoing	___	___	___	___	___
Novices					
Class	___	___	___	___	___
Clinical	___	___	___	___	___
Meetings	___	___	___	___	___
Clerical Time	___	___	___	___	___
Other ___					

Total ___

OPERATING COST	Projected Cost (Cur. Prices)	Inflation Factor	Final Estimated Cost
Books	___	___	___
Periodicals/subscriptions	___	___	___
Dues/membership fees	___	___	___
Med/Surg supplies	___	___	___
Clerical supplies	___	___	___
Repairs and maintenance	___	___	___
Legal and professional fees	___	___	___
Consulting fees	___	___	___
Education:			
Travel	___	___	___
Tuition/registration	___	___	___
Consultation/speaker fees	___	___	___
Audiovisual supplies	___	___	___
Publicity	___	___	___
Printing	___	___	___
Other: ___	___	___	___
___	___	___	___

Total ___

Exhibit 3-4 continued

CAPITAL EXPENSES	Proj. Cost	Inflation Factor	Est. Cost
Audiovisual	————	————	————
Equipment	————	————	————
Programming	————	————	————
Medical surgical equipment	————	————	————
Other: _____	————	————	————
_____	————	————	————
_____	————	————	————
		Total —————	
		Final Total —————	

to examine materials already available within the facility or on the market. If these can be adapted or used "as is", you will save a considerable amount of time. Multiply the number of hours by the cost per hour of the persons involved.

Operating and Capital Costs

Once manpower costs have been calculated, the next step is operating and capital expenses. To determine operating expenses, one needs to project the cost of supplies and the day-to-day expense of doing business. Such items as books, periodicals, subscriptions, dues and membership fees, medical, surgical, and clerical supplies, repairs and maintenance, and legal and professional fees may be included. Be sure to plan for recreational activities, such as birthday or holiday celebrations, if that is appropriate. Remember also to include the cost of inflation in your projections. Most institutions have set percentages they use to plan for inflation.

Capital expenses are costs for major equipment and supplies, generally over some set amount, such as $100.00. List the equipment that will fall into this category; then calculate its price. Consult your purchasing department if assistance is needed in determining prices. Finally, total your figures. This is your projected budget for the period of time you identified. If it comes to a great deal more than you expected, trim things down or anticipate where cuts might be made if necessary.

Write Performance Descriptions

The next preparatory step for the program is the writing of performance descriptions. Job descriptions, as they are often called, are specific definitions of the duties and responsibilities of a position. They explain in detail the required or expected behaviors.

Well-written job descriptions are important. They define behaviors expected of the person in particular positions and are the basis for evaluation. Sloppy or vaguely written descriptions confuse everyone and are worse than having none at all.

In many cases, writing job descriptions will be unnecessary. Your program will utilize the existing organizational descriptions. Examine these to be sure that expectations are clearly defined but avoid the time-consuming task of re-writing whenever possible.

In the case of new programs, however, writing job descriptions may be unavoidable. Each position in the program, including administrator, coordinator, instructors (if any), managers, preceptors, and novices, should have clearly defined expectations for behaviors. For the novices, behaviors should be explicitly defined for each particular program. Specific behaviors for the preceptors, coordinators, managers, and administration may be included in their primary job description. For example, the preceptor role may be one component of Level II performance within a clinical ladder. The actions and attitudes necessary for a preceptor may be precisely outlined within their job description. It would be duplication to rewrite their job description. Likewise, behaviors needed for administration may be included in the job description of Director of Nursing Education. If administration of the program is not their sole responsibility, a specific job description will need to be written. In some instances, guidelines for performance may be a sufficient adjunct to present job descriptions. Regardless of approach, expectations and responsibilities must be clearly defined and understood by all program participants and staff.

Almost all organizations have a format that is used to write position descriptions. Follow the format of your particular organization, being sure to include the behaviors you feel are necessary for the particular position. Exhibits 3-5 and 3-6 provide examples of job description formats and performance guidelines.

Determine Evaluation Procedures

The next step in the planning process is the determination of evaluation methodologies. We will discuss methods and the setting up of a personnel evaluation system but will defer the giving of evaluations until Chapter 13.

Personnel appraisal systems provide a forum for determination of progress. They facilitate feedback, diagnosis of strengths, analysis of needs, and planning for improvement. Although often considered traumatic for both manager and employee, evaluation can be a positive experience. Periodic appraisal of progress toward objectives or goals is essential if one is to know how one is doing.

Exhibit 3-5 Job Description Format

Job Title:

Overview of Position:

Functions:

Requirements and Qualifications:

Position Relationships:*
  Supervised by:
  Persons supervised:
  Promotion to:
  Promotion from:
  Comments:

  *Adapted from position descriptions used at Providence Hospital, Everett, Washington.

Exhibit 3-6 Preceptor Guidelines

Preceptors are responsible for:

1. Reviewing self-assessment forms before the novice begins.
2. Reviewing clinical skills list with the novice when the novice begins on the clinical unit.
3. Acting as a teacher, resource person, and clinical role model for the novice.
4. Coordinating learning experiences for the novice, including times when the preceptor will be absent from the unit.
5. Providing ongoing support and feedback to the novice.
6. Validating skills and updating the clinical skills list.
7. Writing evaluations, sharing them with the novice, and submitting them to the program coordinator.
8. Contacting the program coordinator for problems or difficulties with the novice.

Effective Appraisals

Effective performance appraisals have several characteristics. Clear expectations are set, the objectives and purpose of the program are communicated, and a standard of performance for the position is clearly established.

The purpose of the appraisal must be identified, communicated, and understood by those who will participate in it. A coaching and counseling approach should be adopted, concentrating on what can be done to improve performance, rather than focusing on the negatives of past performances.

The process of the evaluation must be considered fair and productive by participants. If appraisals are seen as partial to or favoring a selected few, or if they are considered a waste of time, little will be gained by either the appraiser or the appraisee.

Numerous decisions must be made in designing a system that works effectively.

What Criteria Should Be Used?

Personnel appraisal may be either normative or criterion based. Normative-referenced evaluation compares one individual's progress or achievement with that of others. These others may be additional novices within the program at the same time, novices from previous programs or institutions, or established norm groups. Criterion-referenced evaluation compares an individual's achievement with predetermined standards.

The choice of one system over another depends on the desired outcome. As Bevis (1978) explains it:

> If the teacher is trying to determine whether or not the behaviors deemed necessary to the intent of the course have been achieved, the choice will be criteria performance methods. If, on the other hand, the teacher desires a point of reference for determining how a student is performing in relation to other students (either in the same class, in other sections of the class, or in other nursing programs), norm performance methods are indicated. (p. 193)

The criteria to be used for evaluation should be based on the written goals and objectives of the program and reflect the novice's progress or lack of progress toward those goals.

The preciseness of learning objectives is crucial. If those objectives are clear and concise, measurement of attainment is relatively easy. If objectives are vague or imprecisely written, measurement will be difficult or impossible.

Criteria must be understandable. They should be written in language that will be familiar to both the person doing the appraisal and the one being appraised. In order to minimize confusion, only one aspect of performance should be addressed at a time.

Measurability is also important. Criteria should be specific and as objectively quantifiable as possible. For example, "understands medication procedure" is difficult to measure or quantify; "demonstrates correct hospital procedure for administration of medications" is both finite and measurable.

Criteria must be behavioral. They must specify, in behavioral terms, what is to be learned, demonstrated, or valued. These must be expressed as behavior to be exhibited by the person being evaluated, rather than by others. When criteria are stated as expected behaviors, recognizing achievement or lack of attainment is clearer.

Finally, criteria must be achievable. They must be attainable within the time period allotted and must be possible within the constraints imposed. In other words, they must be related to the program's general goals and objectives and consistent with organizational philosophies, policies, and procedures, and with the resources available.

Who Will Be Evaluated?

It is logical, of course, that novices will be evaluated. But beyond that, are there others who will need to be assessed for their performance? Of specific concern are the preceptors.

Opinions vary on the need and desirability of formal preceptor evaluations. Some argue that such evaluations are only fair—in reality preceptors are being evaluated whether they realize it or not. It is fairer to be open and above-board and communicate the criteria than it is to be covert about the matter. Moreover, preceptors need feedback themselves if they are to upgrade their skills.

Others maintain that preceptors need not be formally evaluated, that the co-ordinator has the responsibility to be sure the program runs smoothly and to serve as a resource for the preceptors, and that preceptors themselves are best able to assess their performance and seek ways to upgrade it. Coordinators can help preceptors do this if they are unable to do so themselves by exploring particular situations with the specific individual. Self-evaluation forms can be used to help preceptors define their level of performance and further needs.

Often, it is best to leave the decision to the preceptors. When they are ready for evaluations, they will ask for them. Until then, it is sometimes wisest to leave the issue unopened; forcing evaluations on preceptors before they are ready for the feedback can be very threatening.

Who Should Do the Evaluating?

Generally, it is appropriate for preceptors to evaluate the novices, as it is they who are working most closely with them and are in the best position to observe performance and progress. Some facilities prefer to have the program coordinator or head nurse evaluate progress, however, as they are less directly involved with the learner and are consequently able to be more objective. While the former is probably preferable, it is a matter for individual decision and depends on your objectives and the particular institution.

If you decide to include a formal evaluation of preceptors within your program, decisions about who evaluates them are less easy to make. There are several choices: coordinators, head nurses, or novices.

Coordinators should be continually evaluating preceptors, albeit usually on an informal basis. To extend this to a formal process is not difficult. Coordinators are in ideal positions to assess preceptor performance. Receiving feedback from novices, preceptors, and head nurses alike, they are able to synthesize a total picture of the preceptor's abilities and needs. As resource persons they are able to assist preceptors in developing skills that are lacking. Coordinators, however, are not usually in positions of line authority above the preceptor and having them write evaluations on only one aspect of total performance may create difficulties by blurring organizational lines.

As a result, many prefer that the head nurse write preceptor evaluations, whether as part of an overall annual or semiannual performance review or as a separate and distinct entity. As far as line authority, the head nurse is in the most appropriate position organizationally to evaluate the preceptor. However, as the head nurse's expectations and unwritten criteria may be different from those expressed for the program, care must be taken that the precepting aspects of evaluation are based on the performance desired by the program.

Finally, there is the option of having the novices evaluate the preceptors' performance. This is, from the preceptors' point of view, probably the most helpful approach. Receiving direct testimony from novices on what did or did not facilitate learning allows the preceptors to reexamine their performance. Techniques that they felt were ineffective may in fact have been perceived by their novices as extremely beneficial, or vice versa. As long as evaluation formats focus on learning techniques rather than personalities, this is usually the most advantageous approach.

How Often Will Evaluations Be Done?

The frequency of evaluation is a matter of personal choice but there should probably be at least one rating from each preceptor at least once a month during the program. Too frequent evaluations become repetitious, making progress slow and dampening motivation; too long a period between evaluations provides insufficient feedback and too little positive reinforcement.

Format

Much of the success or failure of performance appraisals depends on the format used. An appraisal system should be comprehensive, confidential, and easily understood. A variety of methods are available that can meet these criteria. These include essays, checklists, field ratings, rating scales, observation, exams or tests, questionnaires, anecdotal notes and critical incidents, as well as management by objectives (see Chapter 7).

Revise Your Program Plan

Following determination of evaluation methods, the program plan should be revised to reflect the new information and ideas you desire to incorporate. As this will not be the final draft, it need not be flawless. However, this draft is what will be used to secure final organizational approvals, and you will want to be sure that it accurately represents the scope, design, and content of the program.

Secure Final Approvals

Now, secure the final approvals needed to proceed with the program. Be sure to follow your organization's protocol for securing approval. If there are difficulties in convincing key personnel of the program's benefits, refer to the section on marketing at the beginning of this chapter.

SUMMARY

This chapter has examined the process of planning required by the decision to pursue a preceptor program. Exploration and preparation of a program plan are preliminary steps. The next chapter will explore marketing that plan and finding appropriate personnel who will contribute to its implementation.

REFERENCES

Bevis, E.O. (1978). *Curriculum building in nursing: A process* (2nd ed.). St. Louis: Mosby.

Ferris, L. (1980). Cardiac preceptor model: Access to learning by nurses in rural communities. *Journal of Continuing Education in Nursing, 11*(1), 19–23.

Kotler, P. (1972). *Marketing management: Analysis, planning, and control* (2nd ed.). Englewood Cliffs, NJ: Prentice-Hall.

Selg, M.J., & Morrow, K.L. (1981). *Graduate nurse residency program: Plan IV*. Everett, WA: Providence Hospital.

Chapter 4

Finding Appropriate Personnel

A completed plan will be a final, polished version of your program with all facts and descriptions accurate and format and typing flawless. The plan presents, both in appearance and content, the image you desire to convey. (Appendix C is an example of a complete program plan.) Once the plan has been finalized, you can move into marketing of the program and selecting the personnel that will make it work. That is the subject of this chapter.

In reality, as we have seen, internal marketing is an integral and vital part of the planning process. The program must be successfully marketed throughout the planning process if it is to prosper.

Marketing is important to all organizations that seek to serve and satisfy specific publics. Just as hospitals seek to satisfy physicians, staff, and patients, so must specific departments or programs seek to satisfy their specific publics.

Preceptor programs serve a diverse public that includes administration, novices, users of the program's "product," preceptors, and so forth. There is even a general public, in that persons outside the organization, such as potential novices and school faculties, must often be sold on the worth of the program.

We have already discussed internal marketing. What are some methods for external marketing? Obviously, word of mouth from satisfied novices will be a strong marketing aid and should be supported and encouraged whenever possible. There are, however, other techniques that deserve investigation.

RECRUITING

Consider including references to your program in your job advertisements. Such references will stimulate interest in your program among job applicants, bring persons interested in your program to your institution, and raise awareness of your program among professional colleagues. Many nursing managers and educators read the help wanted advertisements to keep up with the market in their community. In addition, this is often inexpensive advertising as ads are routinely placed in efforts to fill vacant positions.

Be sure your own staff is aware of the program. Occasionally, we become so caught up in our own corner of the world that we neglect the obvious. Members of the general staff, other departments as well as nursing, can be very effective in spreading information about the program to friends and colleagues outside the facility. To do so, however, they must be aware of the particular program and somewhat familiar with its content and intended audience. At the least, they must know who the program's contact person is. Use the methods commonly employed in your organization (staff meetings, notices, memos, newsletters, etc.) to spread the word. It usually pays off.

Use recruitment affairs whenever possible. Include a one-page description of the program in the packets sent or handed out to prospective employees, for example. (See Exhibit 4-1 for one example.) Be sure persons knowledgeable about the program are at recruitment booths. Offer speakers to local schools of nursing on related topics—"What to look for in new graduate residency programs," for example. The opportunities are unlimited.

Consider also professional gatherings and meetings. Many such meetings have a general "sharing" time used to bring everyone up to date with what's been happening. Share your excitement and enthusiasm for the program at these events. The more people who know of the program, the greater the potential for referrals.

Consider publishing. Many journals are interested in articles detailing new programs or solutions to problems. Such ventures will bring you broader recognition and contribute to overall knowledge about the program's existence.

The opportunities are endless, and have barely been touched on here. Although it is possible to spend large amounts of money, the methods included here are all relatively inexpensive. Successful marketing doesn't depend on cost—it is limited only by your imagination.

THE SELECTION PROCESS

The next major job is the selection of program personnel. There are two reasons to be selective about the people you hire. First, you increase the chances for success if you hire the type of people needed. They must be capable of performing the activities that need to be done, or you doom your endeavors at their conception. Second, people are the crucial element in any effort. Unless you have the kind of people who can not only do the job but also successfully interact with others, difficulties are bound to ensue. The selection process involves several steps. These include defining the qualities that are important for the successful candidate to possess, selecting a methodology, and, finally, conducting the actual interview and choice of one candidate over others.

Exhibit 4-1 Graduate Nurse Residency Program

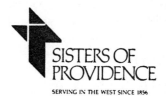

PROVIDENCE
HOSPITAL

SISTERS OF
PROVIDENCE

PACIFIC & NASSAU
P.O. BOX 1067
EVERETT, WASHINGTON 98206
PHONE: (206) 258-7123

SERVING IN THE WEST SINCE 1856

GRADUATE NURSE RESIDENCY PROGRAM
PROVIDENCE HOSPITAL

PURPOSE: To provide an extended clinical experience for the graduate nurse in preparation for assuming the role of a Registered Nurse in an acute health care facility.

LENGTH OF PROGRAM: 11 or 13 Weeks

FREQUENCY: Flexible starting dates

SALARY: To begin, will be Graduate Nurse Non-Licensed.
Following successful completion of State Boards, will be Graduate Nurse licensed.
Following completion of program, will be Base scale R.N.

BENEFITS: Following completion of the 11/13 week program, the resident will be eligible for the following benefits:

Medical, dental and life insurance
Holiday pay
Sick time and vacation accrual from date of hire

JOB PLACEMENT: Following successful completion of the program, the Resident may apply for any open position in the acute medical-surgical units (including Peds and Rehab).

APPLICANTS: From accredited school of nursing; able to identify own learning needs and to prepare independently for the kinds of patients they will be caring for during program. They assume schedules of assigned preceptor(s), and must be able to work all shifts during residency and until a permanent position is found. A resident who fails to receive permanent licensure will be dropped from the program.

SELECTION: By the Associate Director of Medical-Surgical Nursing on the basis of personal achievement in nursing school, professional attitude toward nursing and goals for the Residency Program. References will be contacted.

IF INTERESTED: Submit application or apply in person at Personnel Department, Providence Hospital, Pacific & Nassau (P. O. Box 1067), Everett, Washington, 98206 (258-7561).

Source: Providence Hospital, Everett, Washington. Used with permission.

Determining Qualifications

Certain attributes are needed for each of the positions envisioned. For preceptor programs these attributes cluster in the clinical, interpersonal, leadership, professional, and teaching realms. Let us look at each of the roles separately.

Program Coordinator

First, establish the desirable attributes of the program coordinator. This person is in a key role, as coordination between all elements of the program is essential. Areas of skill to consider as qualifications for a program coordinator include clinical expertise, interpersonal skills, leadership ability, professional attitude, teaching ability, and commitment.

Whether or not the coordinator is expected to teach clinical skills, clinical expertise is a necessity. The coordinator must have had the opportunity to practice those skills in the real setting, and to learn the "tricks of the trade." Without this experience, credibility is difficult or impossible to achieve. So also will be an understanding of the frustrations inherent in the role the novices are learning. In order to offer the necessary support to both preceptors and novices the coordinator must have a solid clinical background.

Leadership ability is, of course, a necessity. The person who assumes a coordinator role will be responsible for drawing together diverse elements within the program and for helping to set future directions. Coordinators are responsible for the day-to-day implementation of the program. Without skillful leadership the program will flounder. This requires patience, flexibility, and a high tolerance level. There will probably be as many precepting styles as there are preceptors.

Interpersonal skills are a requirement for anyone working with others. This is one of the main responsibilities of the coordinator. All factions within the program must be working together to accomplish the desired end. Skills in motivating people, handling conflict, and effective communication are all indispensable.

A professional attitude is an essential as well. The preceptors, as well as the novices, will look to the coordinator as a role model for behaviors. A nonprofessional attitude quickly affects all aspects of a project and will ultimately threaten what you hope to accomplish.

The ability to teach is imperative. This does not mean that coordinators must be experts at classroom instruction. It does mean that they must be skilled in the informal, one-to-one instruction from which we learn the majority of our information. Without the ability to impart new information effectively to novices, preceptors, and managers alike, the coordinator will probably fail.

The final, and probably most important, requirement for coordinators to possess is commitment to the preceptor concept and to your program. The person who assumes this role must be convinced of the worth of the program, and must be willing to spend time and energy to support it. During the first or second runthrough of the program it is particularly essential that the coordinator not be planning to leave the facility. Much of the impetus of the program will be lost if that occurs.

Preceptors

While coordinator selection is important, selection of appropriate preceptors will be the most crucial decision in the entire program. Preceptors determine the program's success or failure, as they are the persons who must implement its objectives. Four areas stand out as being of paramount importance in selecting preceptors: clinical expertise, interpersonal skills, teaching and leadership ability, and professional attributes. The type of novice you are preparing and their level will determine which areas you consider most important.

Clinical expertise is essential for most preceptors. Clinical practice is usually the basis for everything the preceptor does. Preceptors-to-be should be skilled in the use of the nursing process and should demonstrate an ability to apply that process in both routine and complex nursing situations. Decisions should be deliberate and thoughtfully based on scientific and behavioral principles and thorough assessments. Preceptors should be sensitive in their dealings with patients, employing the "art" as well as the science of nursing. Potential areas of exploration include patient teaching, knowledge and use of resources, the ability to sustain and support the patient, and expertise in both basic and advanced nursing skills. Without the ability to safely and appropriately plan, deliver, and supervise care the preceptor will not be effective. Clinical expertise may be extended to include those skills needed for the job: e.g., management skills rather than patient care skills would be the focus of interest for management preceptors.

Interpersonal skills are also important to the preceptor. The ability to promote positive interpersonal relationships through tactful, patient, direct, and sensitive interaction is crucial, and is basic to precepting. The willingness to work with and provide both positive and negative feedback to the novice is a decisive factor in selection. No matter how high the level of clinical expertise, if potential preceptors are not willing to undertake the task of providing negative as well as positive feedback they will never be effective as preceptors.

Leadership and teaching skills are also essential attributes for potential preceptors. They are combined here because they are so closely entwined within the preceptor's role. Leadership means the demonstrated ability to set priorities, to make sound decisions, and to take the risks needed to obtain what is needed. Without these attributes the preceptor cannot provide the desired role model.

Teaching skills are, of course, important, as preceptors are actively involved in the instruction of their novices. Such skills include identification of learning needs in conjunction with the novice, the planning and accomplishment of activities to meet those needs, and evaluation. The skillful staff nurse already displays many of these behaviors in patient teaching and in interactions with new staff or students on the clinical unit. Preceptors introduce and interpret protocols, policies, and procedures and assist learners to build the skills necessary for effective functioning on the unit. Here again, a willingness to provide negative as well as positive feedback is important for the novice's development. Although growth occurs through positive feedback, negative feedback is essential for indicating what aspects of performance need improvement and how behavior is interpreted by others. Seek out as preceptors individuals the staff already uses as resources and who encourage the growth of others. Persons selected as preceptors must be willing to "let go" of their novices and to encourage and support independent growth if the preceptor system is to be successful.

The final attribute needed by a preceptor-to-be is the possession of professional attributes. This means a variety of things in addition to providing quality patient care, however that is defined within the facility. Preceptors should actively participate in health team activities (patient education, patient care conferences, multidisciplinary rounds, etc.) and show an interest in professional growth through participation in learning activities such as seminars, conferences, and workshops.

In addition preceptors need to exhibit bicultural attributes, i.e., to be able to constructively resolve professional or bureaucratic conflicts. Particularly if the novices are new graduates, providing the kind of high quality patient care one has been taught in school within the bureaucratic and busy hospital setting can be one of the most difficult transitions to be faced in an entire career. Potential preceptors must be able to demonstrate their value systems at work within the institutional setting if they are to assist new graduates to develop in positive ways.

Each of these attributes is important. The chances are good, however, that you won't find all of them in "star" quantities in every potential preceptor. Tailor your interviewing questions to elicit information on each of these areas, or enlist the aid of the head nurse or clinical supervisor in determining which nurses are best suited to the role of a preceptor. Remember that it may be possible to develop areas that are weak, and that patience, an open inquiring attitude, and a willingness to support and encourage independent growth in others can be the decisive factors.

Novices

Finally, one must consider selection of the novices. Clinical and educational background, interpersonal skills, aptitude, and capabilities are areas to be explored. The type of program you are beginning and the end product you desire determine which of these areas carries more importance. Chapter 5 discusses novice selection in more detail.

Having defined the attributes and qualifications you seek, you now need to find the right person for the job. Selecting the right person for a job is one of the most important things you can do. Selecting the wrong person can be disastrous and leads to endless headaches.

What course, then, should the selection process follow? The fundamental step, of course, is an initial contact. The normal form of advertising for your facility should be pursued. This often means that the position is posted within the facility for a given period of time, and in-house candidates are interviewed. If no suitable candidate is found, the position is then advertised on the open market. Once suitable candidates are located, interviewing can begin.

Interviewing

There are several interviewing techniques and, for the most part, choice of one over another is a matter of personal preference and institutional guidelines. Three methods—the subjective, point system, and consensus—will be discussed here.

Subjective selection methods rely on the assessment and intuition of the interviewer. Selection is based solely on personal choice. No objective criteria per se are utilized, nor, usually, is more than one person involved in the choice. This system generally works remarkably well. The interviewer often has a precise idea of the type of person who could do the job and the personality that will mesh with the department and the organization. Occasionally, however, personal predilections prejudice the outcome.

Another method of selection is the point system. Interviewing questions are predetermined by one or several persons and points are assigned for each question. The same questions are asked of all candidates and at the end of the interviews points are tallied. The candidate with the most points is offered the position. This method works well because it removes some of the subjectiveness from the interviewing process. However, it is often difficult to objectively document intangibles that you feel qualify one applicant over another.

The third method is that of a consensus opinion. In this method several interviewers converse with the candidate, either serially or in a group setting. Frequently, an initial screening interview is followed by one or more interviews with key people. At the conclusion, the group decides together on the best candidate. In some instances, a point system is utilized. This system works well because the decision is shared by several people and an individual interviewer is less likely to be swayed by personal dislike. Difficulties sometimes arise, however, when opinions are divided between two or more candidates and an impasse is reached.

Each of these methods has its own advantages and drawbacks. The choice of one over another lies solely in individual preference and organizational policy.

Regardless of their differences, all methods are concerned with looking for the candidate with the qualifications, ability, and willingness to do the job.

Interviewing is a skill that improves with practice. The more practice, the better one becomes at drawing out the information needed. Some basic guidelines are presented in Exhibit 4-2.

Content and Context

It is imperative that the interviewer prepare before the interview is conducted. Both the content and context of the interview need to be decided. If either of these is missing, you will fail to achieve the objective of gathering the right information.

Content is defined as the topics to be covered. The interviewer will want to know the applicant's educational background, past work experiences, and personal interests. From the answers, an impression of the person's general attitudes and skills will be gained.

Exhibit 4-2 Dos and Don'ts for Interviewing

DOS	DON'TS
Prepare yourself before the interview.	Go in cold.
Allow sufficient time.	Be too brief or superficial.
Provide privacy.	Permit interruptions.
Set the applicant at ease and establish rapport.	Deliberately set out to stress the applicant.
	Do too much talking yourself.
Ask open-ended questions.	Ask nonrelevant questions.
Be clear about the information you want and go after it.	

A NOTE OF CAUTION

Antidiscriminatory legislation has become progressively stricter in recent years. Inquiries in the following areas may be potentially discriminatory.

Citizenship	Race/Color/National Origin
Sex	Name and address of relatives
Religion	Job or job title of spouse
Age	Age and number of dependents
Marital status	Child care arrangements
Height or weight	Arrest record
Physical handicaps	Qualifications not directly related to the job
Military liability	

Check with your personnel department or librarian for specific information pertaining to antidiscriminatory legislation before you interview.

Along with content, the interviewer must decide on an approach and style to be taken during the interview. Many times a semistructured approach is best. General topics and objectives are decided before the interview, but the order and flow of the interview remain flexible. This allows the opportunity to follow up and focus on particular areas of interest yet ensures that all topics will eventually be covered. Exhibit 4-3 lists commonly asked questions for job interviews.

The context in which the interview is conducted is as important as the content covered. Context refers to the way in which the interview is conducted. It includes such items as the environment in which the interview is conducted, the mood set, and communication styles.

Immediately before the interview the interviewer should review the resume or application, scanning it for particular areas of interest or potential exploration. Specific questions and qualifications for the position should be kept in mind during the interview.

The interviewer must be concerned with the environment in which the interview takes place. Privacy is essential to an effective give-and-take between the interviewer and applicant. If complete privacy is unobtainable, as secluded a space as possible should be created by positioning chairs to permit an aura of solitude. Interruptions should be kept to an absolute minimum.

Exhibit 4-3 Commonly Asked Questions for Job Interviewing

- Tell me about your last position (schooling).
- What was your reason for leaving your last position?
- What did you particularly enjoy about your job (school)?
- What did you enjoy less?
- What would you like to be doing five years from now?
- Why are you interested in our organization? The position?
- Describe your definition or philosophy of nursing.
- What do you see as unique to the role of the professional nurse?
- What were some of the problems you encountered in your previous job (schooling) and how did you solve them?
- In general, how would you describe yourself?
- What do you consider your particular strengths?
- In what areas would you like to develop?
- How do you think your supervisors (teachers) would describe you?

Conducting the Interview

Once content areas and a suitable environment have been established, interviewers can turn their attention to the actual interview. This normally follows a pattern of initiation, listening, focusing in, and answering questions.

Initially, the interviewer must set the applicant at ease and establish rapport. While idle chitchat is generally counterproductive, general comments such as "Did you have any trouble finding us?" can serve as an ice breaker and allow a few moments of settling in. A natural, friendly, and sincere approach will do much to set the applicant at ease and promote rapport. The interviewer can then proceed to the general topics that have been outlined.

Active listening during the interview is essential. Ask open-ended questions and let the applicant freely express himself or herself. Try not to be thinking of your next question as the applicant is talking, but pay full attention to the discussion. If you are well prepared, active listening is easier and short notes can quickly be jotted down on topics you may want to pursue later in the interview.

Don't be afraid to take notes during an interview. Although some interviewers believe this detracts from personal give-and-take, it is difficult to remember answers for any length of time, particularly if there are more than a few candidates. Ask candidates if they mind note taking before doing so; few will object if the purpose has been explained.

Also, don't be afraid to delve into particular areas of interest. Although one doesn't want to sharply interrogate the applicant, obtaining specific information is essential if you are to make an intelligent selection. Don't allow the applicant to give too many generalizations ("I left my last position because I felt I couldn't give safe nursing care") without delving into them in depth ("What in particular did you feel wasn't safe? Did you take any steps to attempt to remedy the situation? What happened? Why do you feel they failed?").

In closing the interview, be sure the applicant has the opportunity to ask any questions he or she might have about the position or the organization. Indicate when the selection will be made and how candidates will be notified.

The Decision To Hire

Once the interview is complete and data have been obtained, consider them in light of the position you desire to fill. Watch out for the halo effect, where you assume that if candidates are outstanding in one area they will be outstanding in all; and problem distortion, where a poor performance in one area outweighs positive attributes in others. Remember, the person with the right qualifications, right background, and right attitude is probably the right person for the job.

SUMMARY

When that first notice is posted or you see the first ad in the newspaper, you are off and running. All your ideas, plans, and dreams are in public view. This chapter has described the marketing process and the all-important steps toward putting the right personnel in place. Chapter 5 will bring us to actual implementation.

Implementing Your Program

By now, it probably seems as if the planning process has gone on forever. There are three major areas yet to be explored: preceptor development, candidate selection, and piloting. These will be the subject of this chapter.

PRECEPTOR DEVELOPMENT

As we have noted, preceptors are the key to the program's success. Without successful preceptors a successful program is impossible. Therefore preceptor development warrants both time and energy.

There are five general approaches to developing preceptors: the laissez-faire approach, workshops, classes, self-learning, and a combination of these.

The Laissez-Faire Approach

First, let's look at the "let them get it on their own" method. This is when the department running the program takes no responsibility for training or developing the preceptors and they are left to rely on their own resources. Development occurs because the preceptor is motivated and desires to pursue it. The department may or may not provide the preceptors with a list of resource materials to assist them.

There are several advantages to this approach. Most preceptors are willing and motivated to develop themselves and will search out materials to do so. Since they perceive the need, knowledge gained is more readily applied. Development proceeds at the preceptor's own pace, as needs evolve from experience. Rarely is this the case in other methods as there is normally a group and the pace cannot be set to meet the individual needs of each participant. In addition, experience is often the best teacher; many preceptors learn best what works and what doesn't from trial and error. Finally, this is an inexpensive way to pursue development since it is essentially free, an attractive alternative in financially tight times. Cost may indeed prove the deciding factor in whether a program can be run. The ability to decrease cost by minimizing training expenses may be essential. The coordinator can still serve as a resource and guide individuals in their own self-development if desired.

There are also disadvantages to this method. Preceptors must still function as staff and are therefore limited in the time that can be spent away from the clinical unit. Unless the preceptor is unusually dedicated, self-development may be low on the individual's list of priorities or it may be ignored altogether. In addition, preceptors may not identify the need for improvement on their own and may therefore not pursue needed development in a particular area or areas. This approach also disregards the importance of an institutional commitment to the program and demonstrates the attitude that the expense of developing the program's key people isn't justified.

Workshops

Workshops "provide an active learning experience for one or groups who attempt to explore solutions to assigned topics or problems" (Tobin, Hull, & Yoder Wise, 1979, p. 142). The material covered in the workshop relates to the specific role of the preceptor within the facility and normally includes such topics as the role of the preceptor, adult learning principles, reality shock, communication, evaluations, and the like. Mini-lectures and group work are often components.

There are three major advantages to using workshops. First, they give preceptors the information needed to function efficiently and effectively in a concentrated manner. Most of the material can be covered concisely in a brief period of time. Removing the preceptors from day-to-day responsibilities on the patient care unit allows them to give their exclusive attention to the material being presented and eliminates the strain of trying to concentrate while worrying about patients they have left on the unit. This, of course, enhances learning. In addition, it removes the stress of trying to learn material on their own time with little or no assistance from the institution. Regardless of how dedicated the preceptor may be, it is often difficult to find time to do the compulsory things in life, let alone the discretionary ones.

Second, workshops build rapport among preceptors and promote peer support. This is, of course, not possible in self-learning situations. Often, interchange by group members and the demonstration of mutual support are as valuable as information given by the instructor, and joint problem solving is frequently more effective than anything the instructor could suggest. The program's reality orientation is enhanced by the preceptors' use of fellow preceptors as resources and the chances of it being purely an academic exercise are diminished.

Preceptors, particularly new preceptors, are anxious and feel inadequate in assuming a preceptor role. Concerns center on feelings of inadequacy regarding their clinical knowledge and teaching skills. Mutual sharing of information, solutions, and resources helps new preceptors to deal with these common feelings and to realize that they do have things to offer. In addition, it reinforces the idea that one doesn't have to have all the answers to succeed at precepting.

Third, a workshop demonstrates commitment by the institution. It says, in essence, "We think this program is important; therefore we are willing to spend time and money to make it work and to develop the people on whom its success depends." This demonstration of institutional commitment can be essential to the program's success.

There are, of course, disadvantages to conducting workshops. First, it does cost both time and money. The financial commitment necessary may not always be possible or it may not be feasible to arrange sufficient time either for the instructor to teach or the preceptors to attend. If the workshop is conducted on the employer's time, it is often not possible to arrange for all the preceptors to be off the clinical units at the same time. This leaves you with the choice of not including everyone or of running the program twice—an even more expensive option. If preceptors are to attend on their own time, it is impossible to make attendance mandatory and those who need the material most may not attend. There is also the obstacle of motivating people to come on their own time. In addition, since it is rare for all participants to have their days off on the same day of the week, you may still face the alternatives of having to repeat the program or of missing substantial numbers of preceptors.

Second, one faces the problem that preceptors may not see the necessity for development unless a personal lack has been experienced. Frequently, information is appreciated and utilized if preceptors have faced the problem but ignored if they have not. The preceptor may feel that "I know all that" and it is not until he or she is faced with personal problems in trying to apply the knowledge that the need is acknowledged. This is of particular concern when the individual has not yet precepted at all and thus far sees little relevance in the information being presented.

Finally, there is sometimes a necessity for more information than can be offered within the format available. For example, the material that you plan to present may work out to be 12 hours of content, yet for practical and economic reasons you are limited to a one-day format. This can be particularly frustrating since you are then faced with the choice of overloading the participants or compromising what you feel they need to do the job effectively.

Classes

Another option for preceptor development is a series of classes. Information is presented sequentially in short sessions. This has the advantages of giving the information needed, of extending over a period of time, and therefore providing the opportunity to respond to needs expressed by the group and build rapport among preceptors.

Such a series of classes allows the instructor to provide all the information needed by the preceptors; the time limitation imposed by a workshop does not exist. The full twelve hours of content could be presented in six two-hour classes, for example. It also allows development and progression of material, as one builds on previous content areas and expands them. In addition, preceptors have the opportunity to apply knowledge acquired between classes and a chance for follow-up and clarification during the next session of their class.

As classes extend over a period of time, opportunities exist to have the preceptors define their own areas of need and for the instructor to adapt the classes to meet them. For example, although information may have been presented on writing objectives, further material may be desired by the group on the differences between cognitive, affective, and psychomotor objectives. It is easy for the instructor to arrange for the inclusion of that specific information.

Finally, a series of classes retains the advantage of promoting rapport among preceptors. In fact, classes may be one of the best methods to do this since they maintain a forum for group discussion, problem solving, and mutual support over a period of time. This reinforces the perception of preceptors as resources for one another and promotes opportunities for productive interaction. The peer assistance thus enhances the usefulness of the classes, promotes a reality orientation, and encourages the practical problem-solving approach that ultimately proves most useful for adult learners.

Disadvantages appear here also. Classes may be costly, it often proves difficult to free people from the clinical unit, and individuals may miss classes because of vacations, illness, or the like.

Cost is always a problem. It just may not prove to be practical or feasible to arrange for a series of classes. If a specific time frame is not identified, it may appear as if the classes will continue forever. If a time frame is set, there is the chance that all the needs of the preceptors will not be fully met.

In addition, there is the quandary of freeing people from unit responsibilities. This is actually more of a problem with classes than with a workshop, where the individual is gone for an entire day and can be replaced on the clinical unit. It is also difficult for preceptors to give their full attention to the material being presented. Too often, their thoughts are with patients on the unit and the work that still remains to be done rather than on class content. This limits the productivity of the class.

Finally, there is the difficulty of missed classes. Participants may miss one or more classes because of vacations, days off, illness, or particularly heavy workloads on the unit. This is frustrating for the instructor, who may plan activities for a group only to find that half the number expected attend and that planned activities cannot be completed. In addition, absent participants miss information if the class is held; those who show up suffer if the class is canceled.

Self-Learning

Still another alternative is that of a self-learning resource bank. The department supplies information on a diversity of topics (principles of adult learning, teaching tips, communication, stress management, etc.) in a variety of formats (audio-visuals, readings, audiotapes, and the like). Participants are free to choose the material and form that best suits their needs.

The advantages to this approach are that it allows access to information when the preceptor is ready for it, it allows participants to define their own learning methods, and it allows the participants to define their own needs.

With self-learning the participant acquires information at the time that he or she is ready for it. Learning principles tell us that adults best learn information that they perceive as currently relevant to their needs, yet too often educators fail to provide information at the time that it is wanted by the learner. It is all too easy to provide information at our convenience rather than the learner's.

Furthermore, self-learning allows learners to choose the methods they prefer and have found most effective. Not everyone learns equally well through all approaches; some prefer reading while others find auditory input more valuable, for example. The ability to choose the method preferred helps to enhance learning. Too, since the preceptor is perceiving the need and pursuing the information desired, it is likely that this is the most productive method of supplying information.

Unfortunately, there are some major disadvantages to the self-learning concept. First, the self-learning approach may prove to be quite expensive. Those materials that are on the market are generally expensive and are frequently unsuitable for the particular purposes of this sort of program. One is therefore faced with the prospect of creating what one needs. In addition to the not inconsiderable cost of doing so, the time requirements and lack of available expertise are often prohibitory.

Some persons dislike self-learning materials intensely and on occasion will go to almost any length to avoid using them. Unfortunately, the time and expense involved in a commitment to self-learning often preclude using double systems. Therefore, those persons either ignore development altogether or are forced to seek it in other ways.

Finally, a self-learning approach allows little opportunity for peer exchange. One of its major advantages is that the activities can be pursued at the participant's convenience. This precludes mutual sharing and problem solving, as it is unlikely that all preceptors would choose to pursue their learning at the same time. Self-learning is by definition a solitary activity.

Combining Approaches

None of these approaches is ideal; therefore combinations are often arranged. Two or more of the approaches described above are blended to maximize the advantages and minimize the disadvantages of each. This often works well and potentiates the learning opportunities available for preceptors.

Scheduling

Once the decision is made whether to offer the preceptors a development program, and the type of programming is chosen, one is faced with the question of when the best time is to offer such a program. The options are obvious—before, during, or after the first program.

Pre-program is by far the most comfortable approach for most educators. It follows the logical progression for program planning and provides participants with the most qualified preceptors. Unfortunately, as mentioned above, prospective preceptors may not see a need for the material until it "hits them over the head." This approach also precludes taking advantage of one's own internal resources since participants are not able to draw on their own precepting experiences within the facility.

Intra-program would seem in many ways to be a more practical approach and in some ways it is. Certainly, the preceptors are more likely to see the need for the information and to immediately apply it in the clinical setting. However, it is often difficult to arrange logistically. The coordinator is busy facilitating and coordinating the actual program and the preceptors are actively involved with their novices. Consequently, this approach often proves less than practical.

Post-program? Well—sometimes. Such an approach definitely has the advantage of not interfering with the actual running of the program, the needs are generally well established, and the potential for mutual sharing and problem solving certainly exists. Preceptors would unquestionably be well prepared for the next program. Sad to say, however, the first program's novices would not have the benefit of those well-prepared preceptors. As the first program is probably the most important in terms of the program's life span, this approach may well not be advisable.

What, then, is the best way to develop preceptors? There is no one right answer. The selection of content, format, and schedule for preceptor development depends on the type of program being pursued, its goals and objectives, budget, and the facility's aims, goals, and value system. Any two facilities will find that the right answer for them will be different. Consider the options, and make your choice based on what you feel will work best for your institution.

Content

We have discussed how to present needed information to potential preceptors. Specifically what information should be considered necessary for preceptors? Among topics to be considered are the preceptor's role, expectations for that role, communication skills, role relationships, stress and time management, teaching and learning principles, teaching techniques, the writing of objectives, and performance evaluation. Only a short discussion of these will be offered here, as each of them is explored more fully in later chapters.

First, the preceptor's role and expectations for that role must be defined and discussed. What do you expect of your preceptors? How does that differ from their usual role? What are the rewards for fulfilling or retributions for failing to fulfill the role? How (and when) can they resign if they discover that precepting is not for them? These and many other such questions must be answered before potential preceptors can feel comfortable.

Second, communication skills should have some attention. Successful preceptors must be successful communicators. They must know how and when to communicate and must be skillful in engaging in not only the comfortable communication but the uncomfortable as well. Information on conflict resolution and communicating with difficult people should be an integral part of any preceptor's training.

Role relationships and role building are also an important part of a preceptor's responsibilities and should be addressed in some manner in any development plan. The preceptor must first build a trusting relationship with the novice, and then must assist the novice to build his or her own relationships. Information on topics such as reality shock, for example, will assist the preceptor to interpret and deal with behaviors encountered in the novice.

Stress and time management must be part of a development program. Nursing is an inherently stressful occupation. The additional tension of having a novice dogging your footsteps creates even more tension. In addition, assuming responsibility for a novice essentially reduces the amount of time available for other duties. Consequently, information on both these topics is essential if preceptors are to retain their mental health and effectiveness. Burnout is an ever-present danger.

Teaching and learning principles are crucial to the preceptor's development. Few nursing students are exposed to principles of adult learning in school, yet they are often working almost exclusively with adult learners. Frequently, our teaching is based on the models used when we were in school—with child-oriented learning principles that do not always suit the adult novice. Exploration of adult learning principles and of the importance of self-discovery and timing are essential elements in preceptor effectiveness.

Techniques of teaching are also important. Here again, we base our teaching on what we ourselves experienced—too often the omnipresent lecture. Preceptors need to be exposed to other methods of presenting information, to examine the most useful ways to demonstrate procedures, and to discuss the myriad ways that teaching can occur informally if they are to function optimally.

Preceptors are frequently asked to write objectives or assist their novices in writing objectives. The prospect of developing objectives can be alarming for the person who has never done it. Guidance and instruction will decrease that anxiety and initiate the preceptor into the correct way to set objectives without making it an overwhelming task.

If writing evaluations is an expectation for your preceptors, the methods of doing so must be explored. Few things are as threatening to preceptors as having to write evaluations. Preceptors need information not only on methodology but also on delivery methods, giving criticism and praise, and common reactions from novices.

Almost every institution electing to offer a preceptor development program has chosen to do it differently and to include slightly different information. Appendix I offers one of the many possible workshop designs.

SELECTION OF NOVICES

In many cases, selection of novices will be done by others. Those making the selection should be familiar with the purposes and objectives of the program and keep the program structure in mind when choosing among candidates.

In some cases, you will be selecting novices or assisting in the process. Be sure to specifically identify desirable traits before you begin to interview so that all candidates are judged against the same set of criteria. It may be useful to have the personnel office do an initial screening in the interests of saving time. Be sure the person doing it understands the type of individual and background being sought and arrange to be contacted if there are any questions about the suitability of a candidate. Occasionally, ideal candidates are turned away because of misunderstandings about what is actually wanted or needed.

The ideal candidate will be defined by the purpose and objectives of the program. The interview should assist you to select the candidates you feel will best fit the program and vice versa and to select the best possible candidates for the positions that are available.

Next, the selection process must be chosen. There are a variety of alternatives: committee interview and selection, one individual interviewing and selecting, preliminary screening by one individual, then another individual or group interview and decision. The selection of one alternative over another is a matter of individual and institutional preference.

Guidelines

Selecting potential novices can be a difficult job. There are some guidelines that will be helpful in the interviewing process.

First, set a specific time period for interviews. One to two weeks is generally adequate to interview candidates and finalize a decision. Dragging the process out over a longer period of time serves no real purpose and merely increases tension for everyone.

Leave time before your interviewing period for recruiting efforts. If you advertise that the program will begin on a particular date and let interested persons know that interviews will be scheduled the preceding month, for example, this should be adequate.

Let candidates know the date a decision will be made and stick to it. Nothing is more discouraging for a prospective candidate than to be kept waiting for a lengthy period of time. If it is absolutely mandatory that the decision be postponed, have the courtesy to notify the candidate and communicate the date a final decision will be made. You will quickly lose potential applicants if you gain a reputation for repeatedly keeping candidates dangling.

If qualifications are well defined and you know exactly the type of candidate you desire, consider a rolling acceptance plan. In the normal situation, all candidates are interviewed and a selection is then made based on the best of the candidates. In a rolling acceptance plan, candidates are notified soon after their interview whether they have been accepted, rejected, or are on a "possible" list. Candidates are measured against standard criteria and those who meet the qualifications are hired. This has the advantage of letting potential novices know almost immediately where they stand and of filling positions as qualified candidates appear. It is not appropriate if qualifications are only vaguely defined or if you are seeking only the top percentage of candidates.

Once selections have been made, notify the candidates personally, in writing or by phone. Obviously, the personal approach is feasible in only a small percentage of situations. A phone call followed by a letter is usually the best procedure. This gives the warmth and personal touch needed yet adds the formality to the process that it deserves. It also provides the candidate something in writing to refer to later if questions arise.

PAIRING PRECEPTOR AND NOVICE

Once novices have been offered and have accepted positions, the question facing you is whether to match preceptors and residents. How important is matching? For the most part, one would have to answer "Not very." Nurses learn to deal with all types of persons and this is just one further extension. It will be helpful if preceptor and novice share the same value system—in cases where there is conflict between the novice and preceptor this is generally the cause. However, since the preceptors chosen exemplify the desired value system and candidates are presumably open to that philosophy, this is only rarely a problem. No matching effort need be made if preceptors are skilled.

If possible, however, attempt to match a weak novice with a strong preceptor. To put a weak novice with a weak preceptor will compound disaster. You should not be faced with using weak preceptors. However, there are always those situations where the person you thought would be strong isn't and there is no alternative in sight for the moment. Even if you must rearrange the program for everyone, it is best to do so if the only other option is to leave your weakest novice with your weakest preceptor. If weak novices have the opportunity to strengthen their skills with strong preceptors, often they will turn out stronger than originally anticipated. This will never happen if they are allowed to remain with weak preceptors.

If you feel it necessary to match novices and preceptors, three areas should be considered. These are compatibility, level of expertise, and background. Overall personality often determines compatibility, and it is generally unwise to place two persons who are similar in temperament and outlook together. Some differences seem to smooth the path and promote cooperation rather than friction.

Do not place a preceptor with minimal experience with a greatly experienced novice. (Vice versa is fine.) The preceptor will in all likelihood feel threatened and the novice will wonder what there is to learn from this individual. A match where experience levels are more closely aligned will generally have better results.

In similar manner, try to match novice and preceptor for appropriate backgrounds. For example, it would seem foolish to place a novice with an overwhelming interest in cardiology with a preceptor whose main experience and interest lies in orthopedics, unless it is your intent to expose the novice to a wider range of experiences.

If you desire to have novices use one another for peer support, consider matching novices. This doesn't mean all novices should come from the same program or have exactly the same experiences. They should, however, share much of the orientation, value system, and philosophy of nursing and be willing to openly communicate with one another.

PILOTING

Having selected novices, the next process to consider is a pilot. The purpose of the pilot is to try out the plan and to iron out any problems that have not been foreseen. Inevitably problems will come up that were not anticipated and a pilot gives you the opportunity to straighten out actual or potential difficulties before the program is fully operational.

Content and Length

The selection of a pilot unit (or units) is crucial to predicting the success of the pilot. Do not use problem areas, thinking that the pilot will solve some or all of the difficulties. The pilot needs to be successful; therefore pick the unit or units where it will have the best chance for success. You are trying to prove that your program will work, not that it will fail. Enough problems will emerge even on the best unit for you to tell whether the program has a chance or whether it will never work in the format proposed. That, by the way, is a finding that one must always be prepared for from a pilot; you must consider what alternatives are available if the plan were to fail altogether. Although not likely, the possibility must not be ignored.

How long should a pilot run? Ideally, it should continue for the full length of the program. In any event, it should extend long enough for the initial turmoil of starting up to subside, and for problems to have a chance to surface. Rather than running the program for only a short period of time, consider running it for its full length with only a minimal number of novices—say one or two. This allows the opportunity to fully assess how the program in its entirety will function yet limits the potential for disaster. Candidates should be made aware that the program is in a pilot phase and their cooperation should be enlisted in pinpointing problems and difficulties.

Pitfalls

Once the program is up and running, several pitfalls await the unwary program coordinator. First is an ignorance of the amount of time involved in running the program. Don't be misled into thinking that sustaining a preceptor program is effortless or that the program does not demand further time. A successful program requires time. Preceptors must be carefully chosen and trained on an ongoing basis, candidates continually discussed, and the program reviewed periodically. Trying to do this without budgeting adequate time is futile and results in endless frustration.

Beware of interpersonal conflicts. These can't always be avoided but be sensitive to the potential for conflict and try to negotiate wherever possible. Incorporating others into planning will give them a vested interest in seeing the program succeed. Nothing will ruin a good program faster than ongoing feuds or strife.

Watch out for preceptor burnout. More attention to this topic will be paid in the chapters to follow. Preceptors easily become exhausted in trying to fulfill all aspects of their role. Be aware of this and offer them periodic breaks from precepting. Often, even though preceptors need a break they will be reluctant to tell you so or will not recognize the symptoms in themselves. Encouraging periodic breaks will pay off in the long run.

Be aware of the potential for sabotage. We never like to think that persons we work with would be capable of this but sabotage does occur, either deliberately or subconsciously. When everything seems to be going wrong for no reason, or one area seems to be having an unusual number of problems, consider the possibility. One example of the damage that can occur: preceptor X seemed to have particular difficulty helping her residents spend time at the desk observing the head nurse at work. There were always waiting admissions and patients to take hither and yon. When time was assigned at the desk, the novice inevitably wound up running errands and "helping out" on the unit at the direction of the head nurse. Investigation finally showed that the head nurse saw no purpose to the time spent by the novice observing her role. As a result she found numerous other things for the resident to do that day. Careful explanation of the purpose and continuous reinforcement finally resolved the problem; however, numerous new graduates missed the opportunity to observe the diversity and complexity of the head nurse's role.

Poor personnel choices are, of course, a pitfall to be aware of. Your program can only be as good as the people in it. The best rule of thumb is "When in doubt, don't." Whenever a preceptor or novice is accepted in the face of doubts, regret has almost inevitably followed. If you have that feeling in the pit of your stomach that alerts you to trouble, pay attention to it. You're probably right.

A lack of support by the preceptors for the novices can be devastating. It doesn't happen often but when it does the entire program is likely to collapse like a house of cards. Individual preceptors must be convinced of the importance and worth of the program. If they are not, don't use them in the program. Take the extra time to convince them, or find others. You don't need preceptors who don't believe in the program.

If you do the scheduling, be aware that it can be enormously time consuming and leave sufficient time for it. Establish a procedure and place for requests and set a deadline for them to be in. Then you can be sure they have a fair chance of being granted. Trying to coordinate the schedules of residents, preceptors, and your own work can be an overwhelming task. It is essential that as coordinator you know where the novices are and with whom if you are to be assured that the objectives of the program are being met. Be kind to yourself and leave enough time to do schedules properly.

None of these pitfalls is inevitable yet all can have a devastating impact if they are not avoided early. Awareness is often the difference between a minor problem and a major calamity.

SUMMARY

This chapter has reviewed the final steps of program implementation. It explored the importance of developing preceptors and reviewed several ways to do so. It examined selection of candidates, the pairing of novices and preceptors, and piloting of the program. The next chapter will concentrate on common problems faced by preceptors.

REFERENCE

Tobin, H.M., Hull, P.K., & Yoder Wise, P.S. (1979). *The process of staff development* (2nd ed.). St. Louis: Mosby.

Chapter 6

Common Problems of Preceptors

Until now, we have discussed the planning and setup of a preceptor program. The bulk of a coordinator's time, however, is spent in running the program, particularly in assisting the preceptors to deal with their novices. This is no small job. Coordinators must focus on communication and problem solving as they help preceptors to diagnose, intervene, and evaluate their precepting actions. We shall be exploring the preceptor role in depth throughout Part II. This chapter is intended as an overview.

HELPING RELATIONSHIPS

Both coordinators and preceptors are in helping roles. Kolb and Boyatizes (1974) identify seven strategies that assist individuals to create more effective helping relationships. These are supportiveness, collaborative goal setting, a self-directed emphasis, manipulations of expectations, behavior monitoring, selective reinforcement, and results manipulation.

Supportiveness is directed at creating and maintaining a sense of psychological safety. Such a feeling of safety is essential to psychological well-being and serves as a foundation for learning. An atmosphere of positive regard, empathy, and genuineness will maintain the trust and collaborative environment most conducive to interpersonal relationships. Psychological safety is also enhanced by feeling in control of oneself and one's environment, increased knowledge about events, verbalization and the opportunity to discuss events as they occur, and chances to practice skills that will be needed for mastery of the situation (Nordmark & Rohweder, 1967, pp. 307, 309).

Collaborative goal setting helps to create an effective relationship and is essential for adults. As problem-centered learners, adults react poorly to being told what they need or want. Preceptors and novices must both see the need for information and must assist in setting educative or performative goals if success is to be achieved and if the relationship is to be perceived as a helping rather than a directing and controlling one.

An emphasis on self-direction and self-control is necessary. Adults take personal responsibility for their actions and must make a voluntary commitment to change; it cannot be legislated. The helping role of the coordinator (or preceptor) dictates that we assist preceptors or novices to define their own directions and goals, to integrate and synthesize a set of objectives that encompass needed improvements, and to reinforce their self-control and efforts to achieve their goals rather than imposing our own.

Manipulations or expectations may become necessary. Our attitudes and comments influence the expectations of others. Preceptors and novices must be conditioned to expect success rather than failure. Often novices, and occasionally preceptors, must be encouraged and prepared for achievement instead of defeat. Similarly, expectations for success may have to be tempered with common sense from the coordinator. Occasionally, for instance, new preceptors will expect perfect performance from themselves. As helping individuals, we must assist them to form more realistic expectations of themselves while still retaining positive self-images.

In turn, we must program both novices and preceptors to view occasional failure as part of the learning process rather than as an indication of personal worth. Failures must be accepted as a part of growing. Encouragement to explore, and the absence of psychological punishment for trying new approaches and failing to have them work, is essential. One cannot improve without learning what doesn't work as well as what does.

Monitoring of behavior is essential in helping relationships. Observation and coaching of the preceptor and novice as they attempt to reach their goals are crucial to their success. Feedback and reinforcement of desired conduct and cognition will serve as reminders, stimulate further efforts, and support progress toward the goal.

Selective reinforcement is crucial. We must serve as coaches. Coaches selectively reinforce positive or desirable behaviors. Often they ignore undesirable behavior and thereby extinguish it through neglect. As educators we often do the opposite, reinforcing negatives by giving them our attention. Coaches give immediate, enthusiastic approval of desired behaviors. Educators often give such approval grudgingly if at all. Coaches offer direct, clear, quantitative feedback of the "do the same, do less, do more" variety (Smoyak, 1978). This provides the novice or preceptor with concrete assistance for movement in the desired direction.

Occasionally, those in helping relationships must manipulate results. This does not mean outright deception, but rather focusing on the positives rather than the negatives of performance. Critics reviewing college drama events will occasionally offer such positives as "the makeup was excellent." This makes it possible to lead gently into their real message of "Not so hot, kids." Sometimes, we need to manipulate our reactions or our assessment of the results to reinforce the related positives and forget, for the moment, the negatives.

COPING WITH PRECEPTORSHIP

Helping behaviors must be applied to real situations. The remainder of this chapter will be devoted to a discussion of some of the common problems preceptors face and will include possible solutions or strategies. The suggestions contained here are by no means comprehensive; scores of additional approaches are possible. Hopefully, these ideas will provide a starting place for some individuals and provoke thought for others.

Personality Conflicts

Frequently cited by preceptors as major problems, personality conflicts usually stem from one of three sources: differences in expectations between novices and preceptors, differences in values, and fear.

The first step in handling such conflicts is to identify the real cause of the problem. Sometimes this can be done by the novice and preceptor, but often an objective third party is needed to clearly evaluate and pinpoint the source of conflict. Frank discussions held separately with both parties to identify the specifics of what really bothers each person can usually discover the cause. Active listening is a must for drawing out both facts and feelings so that the preceptor and novice can be helped to find ways of resolving the problem.

Occasionally, novices and preceptors will be unable to recognize the problem or will be uncomfortable in addressing it. Ongoing conflict is unhealthy and cannot be allowed to continue without compromising the outcomes desired for the program. Coordinators must be sensitive to such a situation. If preceptors and novices are uncomfortable coming to the coordinator with such problems, the coordinator must be comfortable in confronting the issue, using a statement such as "You and Sue seem uncomfortable with each other." This often opens the door and gives permission for the issue to be discussed. Once the conflict is in the open, it can be assessed and the causes dealt with.

Preceptor and novice have differing expectations:
Unclear or differing expectations provoke much of the conflict between preceptors and novices. Generally, in such situations the individuals have not clearly outlined what they expect from each other. The result is a situation where each party has an unvoiced agenda for interaction. When they do not meet each other's unvoiced expectations, conflict erupts.

Coordinators who find themselves in these circumstances should encourage both parties to take time out to clarify their expectations of each other. Once the problem has been identified and the preceptor and novice understand the course to be taken, the actual discussion can usually be left to the parties involved. This reinforces your expectations of their adult behavior and of their ability to resolve the problem. Clearing the air and getting down to specifics generally solves the problem.

Differing expectations may stem from a lack of reality orientation by the novice. Preceptors often find themselves frustrated when novices refuse to accept explanations of "real life." Novices, especially new graduates, frequently expect themselves to be all things to all people. Such unrealistic expectations are often perpetuated by academic preparation, which underlines assumptions that nurses must like and deal effectively with everyone. This kind of expectation may be difficult to break if the novice blocks the preceptor's explanations of "real life." Empathetic listening and a supportive atmosphere where the preceptor feels free to verbalize thoughts and reactions may be the best you can hope to provide. Preceptors must be encouraged to let novices progress at their own rate and to provide an atmosphere where the novices feel able to express themselves freely without fear of hearing "I told you so." Providing information to both preceptors and novices on reality shock may be helpful and allows discussion and identification of the novice's present stage of development.

Preceptor and novice have differing values:

Conflicts also arise when the values of preceptors differ significantly from those of their novices. This happens most frequently with an older preceptor and a younger novice; usually when traditional work ethics conflict with more modern hedonistic values. It is important to recognize (1) that this is happening and (2) that neither party is right or wrong. Values are personal; one particular set cannot be legislated. Each party needs to recognize the other's right to his or her own beliefs and values. Once the cause of such a conflict is identified, and each party is able to recognize both his or her own and the other party's right to individual beliefs, such conflicts usually disappear. If they do not, and a compromise working arrangement cannot be reached, an alternative preceptor may need to be arranged for. If this is the case, the coordinator needs to reassess the effectiveness of the original preceptor as a role model.

Novice (or preceptor) is fearful:

Fear is another common reason for conflicts. Frequently fearfulness stems from the misinterpretation of what is expected or the feeling that one should or must know everything. Coordinators can reassure preceptors and novices by discussing their assumptions and expectations with them and by their actions. Discussions between all of the parties involved to clarify expectations will help, as will role modeling behaviors that demonstrate that perfection and a knowledge of everything are not expected.

Organization and Prioritization

Skills in organization and the setting of priorities are important for all professionals, but especially so for clinical practitioners.

Novice is unable to organize and get work done on time:
This is probably one of the most common problems faced by preceptors; it can also be one of the most difficult to deal with.

Encourage preceptors to have patience. Organization and prioritization skills come with experience. Often novices are unclear about the amount of time activities will take or grossly underestimate time requirements. Help both preceptors and novices to set expectations: "This should take you about half an hour because you're new at it. Later, it'll only take you ten or fifteen minutes." Be sure to indicate the amount of time things will take when the novice is learning and how long they will take when the novice is proficient.

Role modeling will help the novice. Encourage preceptors to share their "tricks of the trade" and acknowledge that there are days when all they can hope to do is keep their head above water. Seeing how an experienced staff member prioritizes and organizes time will assist novices in their own organization and prioritization. Even more important than simply seeing is having the freedom to explore the thinking behind the prioritization and organization with the preceptor. ("Why am I doing these first? That's a good question. The reason is that they take longer than the others and we don't want to get interrupted. Since we have time now, I'll get them done even though they're not needed until this afternoon.") The acceptance of questioning and an attitude of open exploration will assist novices to clarify their thinking and facilitate the development of their personal skills.

Don't allow preceptors to set unrealistic expectations for novices. Novices need the opportunity to develop their own systems and therefore need the chance to try various techniques. Some of these will fail and some will be less than optimal. It is frustrating for preceptors to stand back and let novices try things that are likely to fail yet they must be encouraged to do exactly that. If we fail to let our learners try alternatives, we hinder their development and we ourselves fail as teachers.

Novice has difficulty setting priorities:
This and the previous problem often go together. Part of organization is prioritization, as we saw in the example. Novices frequently have difficulty defining what is important or what should come first and why. They need help

in deciding which items need action and which do not, or what is normal and what is abnormal.

Suggest that the preceptor establish a plan of action. Planning before the day begins and periodic checks throughout the day will help the novice to stay on track. Spending a few minutes at the beginning of the day reviewing what is important to do at the moment, what must be done on schedule, what must be done during the shift, and what would be nice but not essential to do (Predd, 1982) can help the novice sort out the myriad activities that must be completed and establish a sense of order. Taking a few minutes at the end of the day to review how things went, to discuss how the novice feels about the day, and to consider where the novice might want to change an approach can also be a useful technique.

Preceptor and novice should discuss the novice's organizational plan together and the preceptor should give gentle feedback if priorities seem misplaced. While some novices may react to this with defensiveness, if approached with sensitivity and in a helping rather than a corrective manner such an exploration can guide novices to examine the thinking behind their prioritization and facilitate improvement.

Noncommunication:

Noncommunication is a difficult problem to deal with. Normally there are few communication problems between novices and preceptors but when difficulties do arise, they provoke frustration on the preceptor's part and intervention by the coordinator is often imperative.

Asking the preceptor to review situations where the novice should have asked for help and did not can sometimes help the preceptor find the cause of the behavior in the preceptor's own actions. If this is not successful, a frank discussion can clear the air. The preceptor must reiterate the expectation that the novice will have many questions and much uncertainty and positively reinforce the novice for sharing thoughts or doubts.

Novice feels threatened by preceptors:
Here again, unclear expectations are often the culprit. However, the precipitating factor is the preceptor's behavior. Preceptors sometimes feel that they (or the novice) must be perfect or that the preceptor or novice cannot share what each is feeling. This leaves the novice feeling threatened.

The coordinator must explore expectations with the preceptor. It is normal that preceptors sometimes feel uncertain or frustrated and they should understand that this will happen. Alternatives and options for reducing the frustration or uncertainty need to be considered. Preceptors need to be reassured that neither they nor the novices are expected to know everything and that you expect them to contact you when they need advice or to talk things over.

Preceptors also need to know that it is acceptable to reveal their fallibility to the novice. It is an intolerable burden on the novice as well as the preceptor when there is an overconcern with perfection. Discussing uncertainty and selecting with the novice the appropriate resource person or the best alternative serves to role model professional, responsible behavior in the best possible way.

Novice feels insecure or fearful:

Some novice insecurity is inevitable and normal. However, when the insecurity interferes with learning, it must be dealt with, and preceptors often need assistance in doing so.

Again, preceptors must examine their own behavior for conscious or unconscious cues they are sending novices. If they are passing on messages that they have concluded the novice is incompetent or incapable of growth, they are inciting the behavior. Preceptors should be encouraged to use positive feedback. This promotes further attempts at accomplishment and rewards the novice for trying. The reward of positive behavior, rather than the punishment of negative behavior, will promote the desired results.

Novice doesn't know own limitations:

The first question must be "Does the novice really not know when help is needed?" If assessment reveals that the novice really does know, then the problem must be reluctance to ask for assistance, either because of fear of rebuke or because the novice is uncomfortable about not knowing all the answers.

If, on the other hand, the novice is lacking in insight and has difficulty determining what he or she knows from what he or she doesn't, your intervention is imperative. Preceptors are not always equipped to deal with this problem, and it should not really be totally their responsibility.

Your approach to the situation must be individualized to match the particular circumstances. A frank discussion with the novice involved is of course essential. Often this provides cues that allow you to assess and determine what the problems and possible solutions are. It may be appropriate to set up a precise program of skills observation and validation or to determine a set of circumstances in which the novice *must* call the preceptor. The solution must fit the specific problem.

Novice doesn't know clinical importance:

Occasionally, preceptors run into novices who do not seem to recognize the significance of signs, symptoms, or test results. While this is obviously distressing, the preceptor must be reminded that this is the reason that novices are novices; they have not yet put all of the pieces into a full picture. Preceptors should be encouraged to share the importance of clinical information immediately and to provide or suggest resource material to the novice as needed. These problems will taper off as the novice becomes more experienced and as bits of information coalesce into a total clinical picture.

Here again, role modeling will show the novice that perfection or knowing it all is not an expectation. The use of resources by the preceptor and the sharing of expertise and alternatives on the part of other staff members will demonstrate far better than explanations that it's okay not to know everything and to ask for assistance.

Preceptor is too busy:

Having too much to do is often given by preceptors as a common reason for noncommunication or lack of followthrough. Time management is crucial for the successful preceptor. Preceptors must be allowed to manage their own time, not let their time be managed by others.

Insufficient time is sometimes a result of overload. Head nurses or charge nurses may decide that as the preceptor has additional help, a heavier caseload can be assigned. While this may be true at the end of the program, it cannot be so at the beginning. Preceptors must be encouraged to share their feelings and thoughts with their management and to negotiate for changes as needed. ("It looks like Mary is going to be a big help to us soon with teaching patients home care. Right now she needs some work with IV and I don't think it would be fair to Mr. Smith for us to assume his teaching right now.") If they are unsuccessful, the coordinator may need to discuss the issue with the managers involved.

Preceptors and novices must be encouraged to set aside time for discussion and evaluation. Caught up in the flurry of daily activities, it is easy to let such matters slide. A set time, such as Mondays right after lunch or each day before the end of shift report, will help to provide a structured time and continuity. Finding a private space or a corner by themselves can also help. Chapter 15 contains additional information on time management for preceptors.

Directions are unclear/One-way communication:

These problems have similar solutions and often go together. Preceptors, in their haste to accomplish all that is to be done, occasionally provide unclear directions or get in the habit of communicating in only one direction: from preceptor to novice. Such communication inhibits full interchange and may be deleterious to both the preceptor-novice relationship and full development of the novice.

Encourage preceptors to start at the basics, assuming that the novice doesn't know about the activity, rather than that he or she does. Also, using open-ended questions, such as "How much experience have you had with chest tubes?" will give more information than questions that allow "yes" or "no" answers, such as "Do you know how to work with chest tubes?" This kind of questioning is less intimidating and it promotes two-way communication. Self-assessment forms or questions can also prove helpful.

Feedback

We might say the preceptor's job is precisely to give feedback. That is the essence of the preceptor-novice relationship. Giving positive feedback is usually easy. Negative feedback, however, often proves more difficult.

Novice's dress or personal habits are not appropriate:
While this issue may sound relatively simple to deal with to the experienced manager, for preceptors inexperienced in giving negative feedback, it is often a very distressing problem. The preceptor faced with an inappropriately dressed novice, one wearing clogs when the policy is no clogs, for example, or one who comes to work with too much perfume, is faced with an unpleasant task. Avoiding the issue, however, will not make it disappear. Preceptors must be assisted to give negative as well as positive feedback and to confront issues as they arise.

Direct confrontation proves difficult for some preceptors. Coordinators should assist these preceptors through active listening, by encouraging them to verbalize their feelings and thoughts, and by assisting them to practice before the confrontation. After listening to the preceptor's thoughts and feelings, have the preceptor identify what action should be taken and how to phrase what will be said. Often approaching such matters from the patient's perspective is helpful: "If I were a patient, I think the smell of your perfume might bother me." Explore tactful and sensitive ways to confront. Role playing through a situation is often helpful to preceptors, allowing them to explore a variety of alternative approaches and to receive feedback on the more effective ones.

If preceptors cannot handle such situations, they should be positively reinforced for what actions they were able to take and the coordinator must handle the direct confrontation. If the coordinator is able to help preceptors take small steps in developing their confrontation abilities, eventually they will be able to handle such incidents themselves.

Novice has poor attitude, is unkind, or says inappropriate things:
Again, preceptors must be encouraged to confront such issues as they arise. The discussion above on dress and personal habits contains suggestions for assisting preceptors. In addition, encouraging or giving permission for preceptors to share their feelings with the novice ("This is how it sounded to me") can help them deal with the issue. Occasionally, obtaining feedback from an impartial third party such as a peer, the coordinator, or the head nurse allows preceptors

to sort out the actual happenings and their feelings. Chapter 14 will contain further information on giving evaluations.

Patience

Primed to value speed and accuracy in clinical practice, the preceptor must be able at the same time to be patient and supportive.

Novice is too slow or too fast:
Novices need time to work out their own solutions and approaches. Providing some guidelines and time limits can help, as can including the element of surprise to decrease the novice's anxiety level. Often, novices who are knowledgeable but inexperienced become tense anticipating events. "Mr. Jones will need a nasogastric tube this afternoon, and I want you to insert it." By the time the procedure is due, the novice is so nervous he or she is unable to do it. Incorporating an element of surprise, "Mr. Jones needs a nasogastric tube. Let's go put it down now," helps to decrease unnecessary anticipatory anxiety and promotes confidence. Preceptors must, however, be sure to allow time for review of the procedure, if necessary.

Occasionally, preceptors do not let novices progress as quickly as they are capable of doing. Hovering or stifling independence frustrates the novice and slows progress. Again, preceptors must be encouraged to assess the novices' level of independence and adjust their style of precepting as needed.

Preceptor needs to let go:
It occasionally helps preceptors just to ventilate their frustrations to the co-ordinator. This kind of "letting go" can ease the tension of having someone dog your footsteps and take vast amounts of time to accomplish minor tasks. Active listening usually defuses the tension and helps the preceptor regain a sense of perspective. (Care should be taken that such airing of feelings does not occur within the hearing of the novice, however.)

It is also helpful to put distance between the novice and preceptor, encouraging the preceptor to let go in another sense. As novices gain increasing skill, they need to work more independently. Periodically evaluating where they are but finding other things to do can help the preceptor decrease the tension and frustration of letting go. This also allows novices to fully test their skills with a supportive resource still at hand.

Dual Responsibilities

Carrying both patient care responsibilities and novice support responsibilities, preceptors may feel torn between the two. The support and caring attitude of the coordinator are essential if preceptors are to maintain their coping abilities.

Preceptor has too heavy a load:

If the issue is one of too heavy a patient care load, the preceptor needs to negotiate with the head nurse or charge nurse. For example:

> Preceptor: "Jane, I noticed you gave Sue and me rooms 200 to 206. This is Sue's first week and she still needs a lot of help with almost everything. Would it be possible for us not to have Mrs. Brown in 206?"
>
> Head Nurse: "There are two of you."
>
> Preceptor: "I recognize that, but Mr. Jones' dressing and Mrs. Smith's hyperalimentation will take a lot of time. I'm afraid Mrs. Brown won't get the care she needs if I'm tied up with Sue in 200 and 202."

This may need to happen on a daily or weekly basis and may require getting to work a few minutes early before schedules are made out.

Other staff feels resentment:

Other staff may need to be educated. This can occur formally, for example, when the preceptor discusses roles and responsibilities at a staff meeting, but it is more likely to be successful if it is less overt. Teaching and explaining within hearing or view of other staff helps to reinforce the value of the additional responsibilities carried by the preceptor.

Sometimes preceptors will return from lunch or a day off and discover that their plan for the novice was completely ignored or that the learning focus for the novice was totally neglected in favor of having some "real work" done. Again, education of other staff members is a key to handling the situation. However, there are some nurses who feel that the attention given to the novice is misplaced, that "we didn't have any of that extra attention, and we did just fine." This attitude is hard to deal with, and rarely will demonstrating preceptor-novice interaction do more than antagonize.

The preceptor should discuss the issue with the novice. Novices in such a situation are certainly aware of the problem and ignoring it won't make them feel any better. They should be encouraged to stand up for themselves and reinforced for being assertive.

If the abuse takes place when the preceptor isn't there, as it usually does, preceptors must plan ahead. They should check schedules and negotiate with another staff member who they think will be supportive to the novice, outlining goals and a plan for the day.

Try to discuss the value of the novice with other staff. Spending time now means that less time will have to be spent answering questions and guiding novices when they are regular staff members; a pool of well-prepared novices means that replacement of vacant positions will occur faster. Discussing the benefit of the novice program with other staff individually can help to decrease negativism and promote a more welcoming atmosphere.

Legal Issues

Preceptors are often concerned about the legalities of precepting. State laws and hospital policies will determine what novices can do unassisted and what must be supervised or cosigned. If you, as a coordinator, are determining hospital policies, remember that the novice will be expected to function as a fully fledged member of the staff on completion of the program and that full patient care or management responsibility should be assumed sometime during the course of the program. Therefore, restrictive policies, such as having every note cosigned, are often counterproductive. Many institutions have no special policies but expect the preceptor and coordinator to assess progress and increase independence of novices as they are ready.

Appropriate Reporting

Novices often have difficulty distinguishing what is important from what is not. As a result, reports or case presentations may be too long or too detailed or too concise and lacking essential information.

Preceptors can help novices by establishing guidelines. Setting expectations for what to include and how long material should be will save everyone time and trouble. General rules such as "if it's on the Kardex, don't include it" help the novice to distinguish critical information. Determining normal from abnormal and significant changes or the important from the routine can also help novices decide what aspects to include.

Consistency is important. Helping novices establish a routine for reports provides a system and a methodical approach that aids in preventing omissions while ensuring confidence that important information is included. Whether a prompt card, the Kardex, or a mnemonic is used is immaterial; using the same order and format will instill a valuable lifelong habit.

Practice sessions may prove a useful way to help the novice. Such sessions can provide the coordinator or preceptor with opportunities for feedback and allow the novice to decide and discuss what information should be included. Taping reports for playback later can also be useful, but then there is no opportunity for improvement before doing it "for real."

SUMMARY

This chapter has concentrated on some of the common problems faced by preceptors and coordinators. The next chapter will consider formats and procedures for evaluating their effectiveness and that of the overall program.

REFERENCES

Kolb, D.A., & Boyatizes, A. (1974). Goal setting and self directed behavior. In D.A. Kolb, I. Rubin, & J. McIntyre, *Organizational psychology: A book of readings* (2nd ed.). Englewood Cliffs, NJ: Prentice-Hall.

Nordmark, M.T., & Rohweder, A.W. (1967). *Scientific foundations of nursing.* Philadelphia: Lippincott.

Predd, C. (1982). How to stay efficient in hectic nursing stations. *Nursing Life,* 50–51.

Smoyak, S.A. (1978). Teaching as coaching. *Nursing Outlook, 26*(6), 361–363.

Chapter 7

Evaluating the Program

This chapter deals with the evaluation of a preceptor program. Personnel appraisals are discussed in Chapters 3 and 14.

As we noted in Chapter 3, plans for program evaluation must be projected long before the program is implemented, not injected as an afterthought. Moreover, evaluation must be planned as carefully as any other aspect of the program, for a great deal depends on its findings as well as the ongoing activities that supply you with data. The need for prior planning becomes obvious when one examines the definition of evaluation. According to Norman (1978):

> Evaluation is the looking back and examining of what we have done, or what we failed to do, compared to the standards we set forth to achieve. It becomes the point of departure for new plans and programs because we were successful; or it dictates we reexamine our planning, and then reorganize and implement again, to take corrective action. (p. 61)

The purpose of evaluation is to stimulate growth and improvement. As Schweer and Gebbie (1976) explain it:

> While educational evaluation performs many functions, its chief goal is to promote continuous improvement in the learner, the teacher, and the curriculum based on evidence discovered through a systematic appraisal. (p. 166)

If evaluations are to be optimally useful, they must answer two questions: "How well is the program performing?" and "What can or should be done to improve it?" These questions cover three areas: problem identification, problem definition, and problem reassessment. Problem identification is concerned with the discovery or confirmation of problems, definition with description or classification of the problem, and reassessment with the determination of the successfulness of actions taken to resolve the problem.

KINDS OF EVALUATION

Knowles (1973) divides evaluation into five types: reaction evaluation, learning evaluation, behavior evaluation, results evaluation, and rediagnosis of learning needs.

Reaction evaluation measures how well participants liked the program. It may examine feelings, perceptions, and subjective reaction but it does not look at whether learning has occurred. Reaction evaluations should be fed back to the program planners before the beginning of the next session so the input can be incorporated.

Learning evaluation looks at how well the participants learned the facts, psychomotor skills, and affective elements that the program attempted to teach. Pre- and post-tests, performance exams, role plays, and simulations can be helpful in examining specific gains.

Behavior evaluation examines specific changes in behavior that occurred as a result of the program. Observational studies by others, process recordings, self-rating scales, and the like may be useful sources of data.

Results evaluation looks at the benefits to the sponsoring organization of the program. These may be improvements in staff satisfaction and morale, cost savings, retention or recruitment, or improved quality of care.

Rediagnosis evaluation determines further areas of learning needs. Androgogical principles remind us that all learning leads to further learning. Rediagnosis helps to define areas of potential improvement or expansion for the program.

In addition to the frameworks mentioned above, evaluation can focus on structure, process, or outcome. *Structure* examines the organizational framework and resources of the program. Such items as the program's lines of authority and accountability, physical facilities, materials, and human resources assigned to the program may be included.

Process examines the program's procedures. This includes how program objectives are carried out and the performance of the program staff. It may also include such items as how faithfully established procedures are followed, how successfully the planning process works, or how adaptable the program is to changes within the organization.

Outcome examines the end results: how thoroughly the program attains its objectives and goals, in other words, the relationship of the finished product to the product originally planned. Whether the product warrants the cost may also be included.

THE EVALUATION PROCESS

The evaluation process consists of several steps: initial planning, establishment of criteria, collection of data, analysis and interpretation of the data, and modification of the program in light of the findings.

After a determination to evaluate the program has been made, numerous planning decisions remain. What is the purpose of your assessment? What criteria do you want? What will be the evaluation's scope? Who will you involve? When will you do it?

First, identify your purpose in doing the evaluation. What do you hope to get from it, or what questions do you wish to answer? Are you interested in reactions, learning gains, behavior changes, results evaluation, or rediagnosis? What specific elements? You must be clear about your goals before you can identify the specific components of the evaluation.

Criteria

Evaluation is directly tied to the program's objectives. For this reason, the preciseness of those objectives is essential. If objectives are clear and concise, assessment of attainment is much easier. If they are vague or loosely written, assessment will be difficult or impossible. The purpose and breadth of the evaluation will determine the depth and specificity of criteria.

Evaluation criteria are specific statements that represent the desired level of accomplishment and identify the degree of attainment to be achieved. Actual performance is compared against that desired level and a judgment made as to whether the program exceeds, meets, or fails to meet the standard. Often, criteria are implicit, i.e., any degree of improvement is acceptable.

Program evaluations must be based on clear standards and must evaluate performance rather than the personalities. Personal characteristics are only important as they contribute to or inhibit the fulfillment of the objectives of the program. In addition, standards must reflect the values on which the program is based and the outcomes desired.

Evaluation criteria must be definitive. Before accepting any criteria as final, it is useful to examine them for several traits. Ask yourself if the criteria are understandable, measurable, behavioral, and achievable. If so, then they are probably acceptable.

Understandable criteria make sense in terms of the program's goals and desired outcomes. They should be written in terms familiar to all who will read them, not in unknown jargon. Do they address only one aspect of evaluation at a time? Do they relate in an obvious way to the desired program outcomes?

Criteria must be measurable. They must specifically identify what is to be learned or achieved. A criterion such as "The program decreases turnover of new graduates" leaves you asking "Decreases by how much?"

If dealing with performance, criteria must be behavioral. Evaluation standards should specify what is to be learned, demonstrated, or valued as expected behaviors. When dealing with purely quantitative aspects of evaluation, such as turnover rates or mean test scores, behavioral statements are not applicable.

Criteria must be achievable. They must be attainable within the time period allotted and within the internal and external constraints imposed. Do they accurately reflect the program's objectives and goals? Are they consistent with the organization's goals, philosophies, policies, and procedures, and with the available resources?

While helpful as a means of clarifying thoughts and goals, it is not always necessary to explicitly detail evaluation criteria. It would be difficult to determine criteria for reaction evaluations, for example, as such evaluations are meant to ascertain the participant's personal response to the program or educational offering. Setting an arbitrary standard of acceptance, e.g., 80 percent of participants found the program helpful, may be less useful than examining the comments and impressions, incorporating suggestions or solutions into the next program, and seeing how the evaluations change. However, as each group consists of different individuals with different values, needs, and experiences, care must be taken not to assume that changes in results are due purely to changes made in the program.

In other situations, it is imperative that evaluation criteria be explicitly outlined. It would be impossible, for example, to compare changes in learning (assessed by a pre- and post-test) without a specified degree of attainment to be achieved. Similarly, results evaluation usually requires explicit, objective determinations of changes, e.g., turnover of new graduates enrolled in the program decreases 20 percent from the rate of those not enrolled.

Statistics

An important prerequisite to program evaluation is the keeping of accurate statistics for your program. Such statistics address the quantitative aspects of your program. How many novices do you take and how often? What is the attrition rate? How many preceptors do you use? Exhibit 7-1 presents a general form for keeping program statistics. Accurate statistics give you the basis for future planning and assist you in putting together an overall picture of what is happening within the program. Such statistics can also provide supporting evidence for identifying needs and planning future programming.

Content

The scope of an evaluation may range from being broad and general to being narrow and specific. The program as a whole may be included or only selected

Exhibit 7-1 Preceptor Program Statistics

PRECEPTOR PROGRAM STATISTICS

	JAN	FEB	MAR	APRIL	MAY	JUNE	JULY	AUGUST	SEPT	OCT	NOV	DEC	19__
Number of Novices													
Number of Preceptors													
Number of Units Involved													
Novices who left prior to end of program (Turnover)													
Hours: Class													
Clinical													
Total													
Cost: Instructors													
Coordinator													
Preceptors													
Novices													
Materials													
Total													

pieces examined. Information on program effectiveness, efficiency, cost effectiveness, or manpower may be solicited. The approach you take will depend on your objectives in doing the evaluation and on the criteria you identify.

Problem identification usually calls for a broader approach; whereas problem definition and reassessment require specific, narrow investigations. While it may be necessary to start with the broad brush and repeatedly narrow the focus until you reach the desired level of detail, examination of selected pieces may provide the needed information more easily at lower cost. For example, a broad general investigation may point up several areas of need. To specifically define the problem one or two further, narrower investigations may be necessary. Finally, a specific reexamination of the problem will be needed to be sure that it has been resolved. However, if the problem is already well defined you may be able to skip the broader evaluation. In addition, it may not be possible or appropriate, for reasons of size, resources, or money to completely examine all aspects of the program concurrently. The setting must be defined. Will you examine all areas used for the program or limit your scope? Depending on the purpose, a single unit may be sufficient to answer your questions.

Whether to include subjective information, objective information, or a mix of both must be decided. Subjective information includes personal reactions, impressions, and the like. Objective information includes things that can be quantified and rationally examined, such as program statistics. Usually, an evaluation will include aspects of both.

When should formal evaluation take place? There are two kinds of evaluation: formative and summative. Formative evaluation takes place during the program and furnishes feedback so that changes to correct or improve the program can be made (Bevis, 1978). Evaluation may be ongoing or it may be stimulated by a crisis, such as a drop in enrollment, a decrease of interest in the program, or an increase in the number of dropouts.

In actuality, much of program appraisal is constant rather than periodic. One receives continual feedback regarding the program, both compliments and complaints. The importance of informal evaluation must not be minimized. To a large extent, this informal grapevine determines the long-term prognosis for the program.

Summative evaluation takes place at the end of a program or program unit and determines if the program goals were met. It assesses the extent and degree to which the desired program objectives and goals were achieved (Bevis, 1978). Several options give you a natural "breaking point": at the end of a unit, such as the end of a shift rotation for a group of novices, when they are to change locations, or at the end of the program.

Personnel

Who should do the evaluating is a value-laden question. You must determine who identifies standards and who completes the evaluation. Who identifies the standards is not really open for debate. Standards are set by whoever designs the program objectives. Evaluation criteria are based on and directly derived from those objectives.

Who completes an evaluation is open to more debate. A frequent controversy among educators is the need for vigorous research techniques in the evaluation of learning programs. While many would argue that strictness is appropriate in any evaluative effort, some would say that only the program's participants can determine if the objectives have been met. Others would argue that only program leaders and instructors are able to assess whether objectives have been met. Still others would insist that the supervisors and managers of the units where the novices have been placed are in the best position to determine this. The more liberal view of Knowles (1973) supports the idea that the participants are the most appropriate persons to evaluate the learning that has occurred and to suggest further learning needs as a measure of the effectiveness of the program. In making your final decision, consider the purpose of the evaluation and select those you feel should be involved. Often it is best to include all these groups to obtain a complete picture. Exhibit 7-2 gives a matrix for determining who should be considered for inclusion.

When considering evaluation, someone always brings up the idea of having the "outside expert" evaluate the program. While this idea may have some validity if your objective is to get help in setting up the process for evaluation, in general it is one to be discouraged. Axford (1969) identifies three principles for program evaluation:

1. Instruments for self-evaluation are preferred to evaluation by others.
2. Program planners should be involved in the evaluation process.
3. Evaluation should be concerned with outcomes and results rather than activities or energy spent.

Ordinarily, the persons involved in the program can do as credible a job, if not more so, than any outside expert. Such experts generally use more time, money, and manpower than is generally available (Popliel, 1977).

Data Collection

Finally, there are decisions to be made regarding the sample. If, for example, preceptors have been chosen as a significant group from which input will be sought, will all preceptors be included? A random sample? Selected units? Include as large a sampling as feasible. Your methods for compiling data (manual or computer) may have a limiting effect on the number of evaluations you can handle.

These decisions may seem overwhelming. The form used in Exhibit 7-3 will help you to define your evaluation decisions; the example outlines the decisions made before drafting an evaluation tool.

Exhibit 7-2 Potential Evaluation Participants

POTENTIAL EVALUATION PARTICIPANTS

Type of Evaluation	Novices	Preceptors	Program Coordinator	Instructors	Managers
Reaction (How well participants liked the program)	For Self	For Self	For Self	For Self	For Self
		←------------If involved as attendee at program------------→			
Learning (Of facts, psycho-motor skills and affective behaviors the program tried to teach)	For Self	For Self or Novice	For Novice or Preceptor	For Novice or Preceptor	Varies, depending on learning being evaluated
Behavior (Behavior changes which occur as a result of the program)	For Self	For Self or Novice	For Novice or Preceptor	Varies depending on behavior	For Novice or Preceptor
Results (Benefits to the sponsoring organization)	No	Perhaps, depending on information sought	Yes	Perhaps, depending on information sought	Yes
Re-diagnosis (Further learning needs)	For Self; can assist Preceptor by identifying techniques which enhanced or inhibited learning	For Novice or Self	For Novice or Preceptor	For Novice or Preceptor	For Novice or Preceptor

Exhibit 7-3 Evaluation Plan

Program To Be Evaluated: _____ *GNRP* _____

General Purpose of Evaluation: *To determine how well the program meets perceived needs of residents.*

Specific Goals/Questions To Be Answered:

1. *Perceived improvement in technical, nursing process, teaching and communication skills, effectiveness of teaching methods/materials.*
2. *Does program facilitate transition from student to professional nurse?*
3. *Program length okay?*
4. *Diagnosis of preceptor learning needs.*
5. *Identify barriers and areas for improvement.*

Scope: *Generally broad overview.*

Setting: *All areas involved in program.*

Type of Information (Objective/Subjective): *Subjective*

When: *End of program.*

Evaluation
Participants   *Novices:*   *All involved in program.*
              Preceptors: *All involved in program.*
              Managers: *All involved in program.*

Evaluation Criteria:

1. *There is a perceived improvement in technical, nursing process and teaching skills.*
2. *Teaching methods are effective for at least 80% of novice respondents.*
3. *Majority of respondents feel transition from student to professional nurse is facilitated.*

Data collection can be either a formal or an informal process. In reality, informal data collection is constant, as persons give feedback on the program and its participants. While this kind of information is invaluable, a more formalized method of data collection guarantees that you hear from all parties involved and standardizes a format, making data analysis easier.

Two aspects to consider in the selection of any tool that attempts to objectively measure achievement are validity and reliability. *Validity* can be defined as the extent to which differences in scores reflect true differences among individuals rather than constant or random error. A rating device can be considered valid when a large percentage of those using it are in agreement regarding each component of the device (Schweer & Gebbie, 1976).

Reliability refers to the consistency of the measurement tool over time, under comparable circumstances. To ensure reliability the tool must produce similar results when different but equally competent raters use it (Schweer & Gebbie, 1976). Exhibit 7-4 gives you a further explanation of these concepts.

The options for data collection tools are numerous. Your choice will be determined by your purpose and criteria.

Tools for assessing reactions exist in numerous formats and styles. Basically, all should ask if the participants felt that the program covered the intended

Exhibit 7-4 Some Important Evaluation Terms

Reliability relates to consistency of evaluation results over different samples of questions, or different raters. Low reliability restricts validity, but high reliability does not guarantee validity. Reliability is reported in terms of reliability coefficients or the standard error of measurement. Reliability estimates vary by length of test, spread of scores of the group tested, difficulty of test, objectivity of scoring, and the method used to estimate reliability.

Validity refers to the truthfulness of interpretations and to the results of an evaluation instrument with a certain population, not to the instrument itself. Test validity can be increased by controlling the following factors: poor test construction, nonstandardized administration and scoring of results, atypical learner responses, nonapplicable validation group, and nonrepresentative behaviors measured.

Content Validity refers to how well the instrument measures the subject content and behaviors being evaluated. To determine content validity, list the major subjects and behavioral changes to be measured, give each a weight in relation to its relative importance, prepare a table of specifications of weights, and construct an evaluation device that closely corresponds to the specifications.

Criterion Related Validity refers to how well the test performance predicts future performance or estimates current performance on some other valued measure. To predict future performance, the usual procedure is to correlate the two sets of test scores and to report them by means of a correlation coefficient. To estimate present performance, expectancy tables are used to show the relationship between measures. A major problem in determining this type of validity is finding a satisfactory criterion of success.

Construct Validity refers to the extent to which test performance can be interpreted in terms of psychological constructs such as reasoning ability and critical thinking. Each construct has an underlying theory that predicts learners' behaviors. Some procedures used to determine construct validity are: analysis of the mental processes required by the test items, comparison of results with groups known to differ on that ability, comparison of scores before and after a learning experience, or correlation with other tests.

From: *The Nurse as Continuing Educator* (pp. 188–189) by Carolyn Clark, 1979. New York: Springer. Copyright © 1979 by Springer Publishing Company. Reprinted by permission.

material or objectives, if teaching methodologies were effective, if personal expectations were met, and what their overall opinions of the program were. Information can be gathered in essays, interviews, discussion groups, rating scales, questionnaires, checklists, or any combination of these.

Tools for evaluating learning also exist in numerous formats. Objective tests (true-false, multiple choice, matching), essays, demonstrations, discussion groups, role plays, simulations, and the like all offer opportunities to assess how well the intended material was learned. Pre- and post-tests are helpful for determining the magnitude of change.

Changes in behavior are more difficult to assess. This requires observers to report actual changes in behavior as a result of the program. Case studies or instructor or preceptor evaluations of participants may also be data sources.

For results evaluation such things as turnover, cost effectiveness, and efficiency may be included. The method used to evaluate results depends on the nature of the evaluative questions asked. Often simple comparisons of before-and-after statistics will be sufficient to answer questions.

Part of results evaluation is an examination of the cost of the program. During the planning phase you identified projected costs. How close did you come? Cost management is an integral expectation for most program managers and an analysis of cost projections versus actual costs will assist you in pinpointing problem areas of overrun and in future financial planning. Exhibit 7-5 gives you a cost analysis sheet and Exhibit 7-6 provides a format for examining projected versus actual costs.

As mentioned previously, a variety of data collection alternatives are available. A few of the more common ones are discussed here.

Organized discussion groups of either staff, users, or novices allow for direct input. No more than 15 to 25 persons should be included (Bevis, 1978) to allow for free expression of opinion from all. Sufficient time should be allowed for everyone to have input, and opinions from everyone should be encouraged. Trust is an important element, and all opinions should be encouraged and respected. It is helpful if a neutral person can be available to take notes, or as an alternative the group leader can list reactions and comments on a flipchart or blackboard. Arrangements must be made to have the information available for reference and use later, however.

Checklists are a common method for evaluation. Such checklists can be used to examine structure, process, or outcomes. They should be based on the program goals or objectives and they should be long enough to cover the desired material but not so long as to be tiring. Checklists are convenient to use and examine. They may be either weighted, where some items are worth more than others, or each item may carry the same worth. Again, they may cover a variety of topics in one tool.

Exhibit 7-5 Preceptor Program Cost Analysis Sheet*

	No.	Class Hours	Total Class Hours	Cost/ Hours	Total Class Cost	No.	Clinical Hours	Total Clinical Hours	Cost/ Hours	Total Clinical Cost	Total Clinical & Class	Cost/ Novice	Comments
Novices	6	40	240	8.00	1920.00	6	400	2400	8.00	19,200	21,120	3520	2wk program 1-wk orientation class 10-wk clinical
Instructor A:	1	4	4	14.40	57.60						57.60	9.60	
B:	1	18	18	10.00	180.00						180.00	30.00	
C:	1	8	8	12.00	96.00						96.00	16.00	
Secretarial		(Prep) 5		8.00	40.00							6.67	
Coordinator	1	10	10	12.00	120.00	1	44	44	12.00	528.	648.00	108.00	4°/wk = Coordination
Preceptors	6					6	400	2400	.50	1,200	1,200.00	200.00	.50=Preceptor Differential
Materials Xerox										10.		1.67	
TOTALS			240		2423.60			2400		20,928	23,351.60	3891.94	

*Cost of fringe benefits not included

Exhibit 7-6 Projected Versus Actual Cost

	Projected	Actual	Difference +/−
Personnel			
Administrator/Coordinator	_____	_____	_____
Preceptor	_____	_____	_____
Novices	_____	_____	_____
Other	_____	_____	_____
Operating Expenses			
Books & Periodicals	_____	_____	_____
Supplies Med/Surg	_____	_____	_____
Clerical	_____	_____	_____
Fees	_____	_____	_____
Education	_____	_____	_____
A-V	_____	_____	_____
Publicity	_____	_____	_____
Printing	_____	_____	_____
Other	_____	_____	_____
Capital			
A-V	_____	_____	_____
Equipment	_____	_____	_____
Med-Surg	_____	_____	_____
Other	_____	_____	_____
TOTALS	_____	_____	_____
	Net Difference +/−		_____

Field ratings are used a great deal in informal settings but are rarer in formal evaluation. Field reviews consist of interviewing others who work with the individual and writing up their comments and ratings. This often happens informally in precepting, as the coordinator interviews the preceptor working with a novice for impressions, comments, and recommendations. Rarely, however, is such information written up or shared with the novice in any but an informal manner.

Rating scales examine a degree of proficiency or acceptability. They provide a standardized method of recording judgments about observed performance. They may be either discrete ("satisfactory," "unsatisfactory") or continuous ("rate from 1 to 5"). Numerous rating scales have been published, and tools such as the Slater Nursing Competencies Rating Scale (Wandelt & Stewart, 1975) may prove useful. Rating scales are easy to work with and understand and can be employed for all types of evaluations.

Chart reviews can be useful in examining problem-solving and nursing performance. While it is true that charting represents only documentation and not actual performance, such reviews can help to point up deficiencies in thinking and logic that all novices are experiencing and to pinpoint deficiencies in the program.

Questionnaires are a common tool used for evaluation. They can encompass a wide variety of uses and are easily constructed and read. They can be designed to solicit reactions, evaluate behavior, and examine results or behavior.

Essays are written impressions in narrative form. Such impressions can be grouped into categories such as program reaction, further learning needs, or learning evaluation. Essays are time consuming to write and read, and are difficult to analyze on any but a subjective level.

Observation answers the questions what was done, how was it done, what was said, when, in what order, where and who was involved (Norman, 1978). Observation is most effective for behavior changes, particularly in the affective or psychomotor realms. Cognitive skills are often difficult to observe and are better evaluated by objective methods.

Objective yardsticks of performance, exams or tests are especially useful for cognitive information. They can be used to assess the affective realm but are poor for evaluating psychomotor skills unless a performance component is included. It is important that tests be written at the level of performance desired, for example, to test problem-solving ability rather than merely recall.

Critical incidents are a variation of anecdotal notes in which a record of all "significant events" is made. This can cause a problem as the evaluator may not be present and may not see all significant events. In addition, there is a tendency to remember and thus record the negative events while forgetting the positive. If this method is to be used, care must be taken to include positive as well as negative events.

Management by objective is another alternative. In recent years, the idea of managing personnel by their own defined objectives has received increasing attention. With this method, individuals define their objectives for a set period of time and are then evaluated for their achievement of their own objectives. This has the advantage of being based on the individual's expressed goals and of not having any hidden agendas. However, care must be taken to include the supervisor's perspective when setting objectives as well as the individual's. This system is often incorporated into preceptor programs and novices can set their own particular goals and objectives within wider program objectives.

Anecdotal notes describe in narrative form observed situations, including what was said or done. While anecdotal notes provide the greatest opportunity to capture significant details, such notes are time consuming and open to individual interpretation. To be useful, an accumulation of notes over a period of time must be made and care must be taken to include positive as well as negative elements.

Obviously, tools that combine these techniques are possible, and are probably more commonly found than pure models. If you are setting up your own personnel evaluation system, and are not locked into an existing system, you are now ready to make some decisions about what you want. Decide the style of format you prefer and which best meets your needs. Before you reinvent the wheel, examine the formats already in place in your facility. Perhaps they can adequately meet your needs or can be rewritten or adapted to meet your needs. This saves you time and trouble. If necessary, design a new format, being sure to reflect the goals and objectives of the program. Appendix G includes several examples of performance tools.

Data Analysis

Once information is collected, it must be analyzed. Such analysis may take the form of a statistical analysis, matrix, or "gut feel."

A statistical analysis is feasible only if the information that was collected is in an objective and numerical format. Descriptive statistics such as the average number of participants per program will probably be of more use than inferential statistics such as the mean, mode, and median of the group unless one is comparing such things as test score results. When possible, computerization can greatly decrease the time and effort required to obtain statistical analyses.

A matrix can be of great use when trying to collate and analyze the results of a program evaluation. Such a format places one set of parameters on a horizontal axis and the other set of parameters on a vertical axis. Results are then filled in within the matrix. Such a format can allow you to easily see trends, strengths, and weaknesses of the program. Exhibit 7-7 gives you an example.

Gut feel, although less than scientific in its approach, can often be of as much use as the other, more scientific approaches. Your reactions, after reading the results of a questionnaire, for example, can give a reasonably clear picture of the program's deficiencies and needs. Many evaluative questions require only a pooling of responses for useful information to emerge.

Reporting Results

The final step in program evaluation is the reporting of information, including both successes and identified problems. Evaluation cannot be considered complete until the information is shared with and accepted by those evaluated. This may include the preceptors and will certainly include the program staff. Action to be taken can then be identified. Such action may include revision or changes to the program, clarification of program objectives, or improvement of instruction.

Exhibit 7-7 Evaluation Matrix

EVALUATION MATRIX EXAMPLE					
Rating:	High Satisfaction	Satisfied	Fair	Dissatisfied	Highly Dissatisfied
Question: 1					
2					
3					
4					
5					
6					
7					
8					
9					
10					
11					
12					
13					
14					
15					
TOTALS					

SUMMARY

This chapter has discussed formats and methodologies for program evaluation. The next chapter considers the application of the information developed in this process.

REFERENCES

Axford, R.W. (1969). *Adult education: The open door*. Scranton, PA: International Textbook.

Bevis, E.O. (1978). *Curriculum building in nursing: A process* (2nd ed.). St. Louis: Mosby.

Knowles, M. (1973). *The adult learner: A neglected species*. Houston: Gulf Publishing.

Norman, J. (1978). The clinical specialist as performance appraiser. *Supervisor Nurse, 9*(7), 62–64.

Popliel, E.S. (1977). *Nursing and the process of continuing education* (2nd ed.). St. Louis: Mosby.

Schweer, J.E., & Gebbie, K.M. (1976). *Creative teaching in clinical nursing* (3rd ed.). St. Louis: Mosby.

Wandelt, M.A., & Stewart, D.S. (1975). *Slater nursing competencies rating scale*. New York: Appleton-Century-Crofts.

Chapter 8

Developing and Expanding Programs

Once a preceptor program is in place, thoughts inevitably turn to improvement or expansion. This chapter concentrates on the development and extension of a preceptor program.

Improvement, or ongoing development, differs from expansion in that improvement refines, enriches, and advances an existing program, whereas expansion enlarges an existing program. Ongoing improvement is an essential ingredient if preceptor programs are to progress and mature; the need for expansion varies according to individual conditions.

There are three basic reasons for development or expansion of a preceptor program. Adaptation to a changing environment may be required, renovation may be sought, or variety and a continuing challenge may be needed for program staff.

Adaptation to a changing environment may become necessary for any preceptor program. Shifts or variations in the political, social, educational, economic, organizational, or administrative climate may provoke the need for modifications if the program is to effectively meet institutional needs. Orientation programs, for example, may have to change as economics become tighter and as fewer new employees enter en masse.

Renovation of the existing program may be needed for a variety of reasons. A successful program will require periodic updating to keep it current or to meet new standards as they are established. A poor one may need remodeling to increase its effectiveness. Renovation may require that additional areas be added to improve outcomes or meet new needs.

A feeling of growth and an ongoing challenge are necessary for retainment of qualified staff, essential, as we have noted, to the effectiveness of the program. Individuals must believe that they possess the requisite skills and that their activities are meaningful. This requires effective feedback from program leaders on the value of the program to its participants as well as on individual performance.

The feedback by itself, however, may be insufficient. New preceptors frequently feel the need to improve their skills as preceptors, and more experienced preceptors may feel themselves becoming stale or apathetic. An environment of learning and growth is essential if staff is to be both effective and challenged.

Regardless of cause, development or expansion of a preceptor program requires thoughtful planning and organization if it is to be successful. Let us first look at improvement, since it is likely that initially your efforts will be directed toward that end.

PROGRAM IMPROVEMENT

Improvement may become desirable because the performance standards for the participants change, because the program is weak in a particular area or areas, or because ongoing development is conceived to be an integral part of the program.

Assessing Needs

Improvement plans must be based on a valid interpretation of where the program is currently and where you desire it to be in the future. A thorough assessment of needs is the first step. A clear-cut indication of necessities within the program helps to determine the scope of activity needed, target areas of specific concern, and assist in priority setting. They generally fall into three major categories: structure, knowledge, and performance.

Structural needs or problems are those that revolve around the ongoing operations and organization of the program. Fiscal resources, quality and quantity of staff, physical facilities, and scheduling are examples. Since these organizational areas may require periodic change or modification to effectively meet the program's needs, they must therefore be periodically assessed.

The two remaining areas concern the personnel of the program. Performance needs or problems stem from a lack of adequate performance *unrelated to a lack of knowledge*. These problems are usually motivational or value related in nature. Such areas as absenteeism, productivity, responsibility, the nature of the job, philosophic differences, and the like may fall into this category.

Knowledge (or educational) needs are defined by Knowles (1970) as a gap between the required and present level of competency. These needs can be met through instruction and training. Such information as the roles and responsibilities of the preceptor, how to write and give evaluations, and teaching techniques are examples.

Having defined the type (or types) of needs you are interested in investigating, you are ready to move on to identification of those needs. Needs can be assessed in many ways. The methods you select will depend on the needs you are attempting to define and the idiosyncrasies of your setting. A complete discussion of specific assessment techniques can be found in Chapters 8 and 9.

Establishing Priorities

Regardless of assessment technique used, there will probably be more needs identified than resources to meet them. Therefore, prioritizing becomes a necessity.

Several factors enter into establishing priorities. Organizational demands, sequencing, current problems, and feasibility are just some of the determinants.

Organizational issues are often the basis for priorities. If, for example, institutional expansion is planned and the primary source for added staff is your program, additions and refinements to your classes may have to be deferred until the current need for additional program graduates is met. Similarly, a need for more cardiac monitors may outweigh your need for more audiovisual equipment.

Sequencing frequently influences priorities. Often, "A" must come before "B" if "B" is to be fully successful. In such cases, it becomes prudent to accomplish "A" before "B," even if "B" is of far greater importance.

Current problems may well define priorities. Particularly if a problem has reached crisis proportions, immediate resolution may be necessary for the health and welfare of the program, its staff, and its participants. For example, before urgently needed changes can be made in the program, the issue of one highly controversial preceptor may need to be confronted.

Feasibility also is frequently a prioritization factor. For example, needs assessment may have identified that a ten-week program would best meet the needs of novices and managers. However, if resources won't support anything more than a six-week program, a ten-week program obviously becomes impossible.

Goals and Objectives

Once needs have been identified and priorities set, concrete goals and objectives for the program can be determined. Objectives may address operational issues (i.e., "Revise scheduling patterns so that no more than one novice is on Unit X at one time"), performance issues ("Preceptors will meet with novices weekly to review progress"), or educational issues ("Novices will identify information that should be included in shift report"). Objectives state in precise, measurable terms what is to be accomplished. As we noted in Chapter 3, specific objectives allow determination of effective implementation techniques, assist in sequencing and coordination of events and activities, and provide a framework for evaluation.

Once objectives have been set, attention can be turned to planning to meet those objectives. For operational objectives, see Chapter 3 on planning. For performance objectives, refer to Chapters 13 and 14; and for educational objectives see Chapters 3, 9, and 10.

PROGRAM EXPANSION

A need to enlarge the program may emerge because additional areas must become involved or because new needs have emerged that require enlarging the current program. For example, the addition of other medical services such as rehabilitation, psych or obstetrics, or a decreasing supply of experienced nurses in the area may prompt expansion.

Planning for expansion incorporates many of the same steps outlined in Chapter 3. You need to secure approvals, seek input from those who will be involved in the expansion, revise the program plan, select personnel, and market appropriately. However, several additional principles need to be stressed.

First, do your expansion slowly. Don't overextend, attempting to expand in all areas at the same time. Minor items and small details will inevitably pose major obstacles. It's easy to be misled into thinking that since the program is doing well in some areas, expansion will be care free. Actually, expansion demands the same type of planning and meticulous attention to detail that beginning a program does. It is often useful to introduce an expansion in the same manner as a pilot, allowing opportunities for changes during the initial stages. Don't rush; a poorly thought out expansion can jeopardize all that you have accomplished.

Be organized and methodical in your approach. Actively involve key people in your planning. At this point, it probably is not feasible to have them change major aspects of the program, but provide choices and opportunities for input whenever possible. It will make implementation easier.

Finally, one note of caution. Don't assume that since the program is presently functioning well it will automatically do well in the new areas. Each situation or area is unique in that the individuals involved are different, their expectations and objectives vary, and their commitment to and involvement in the program will be dissimilar. A preplanned and carefully organized design for expansion will help to ensure success.

PRECEPTOR RECRUITMENT AND REPLACEMENT

Most plans for improvement and expansion of the program require additional preceptors, and inevitably it will become necessary at some point to replace preceptors who transfer to other areas, take leaves, retire, or move away.

Initially, needs and goals for preceptors must be defined. How many new (or replacement) preceptors will be needed and in what time frame? Will expectations remain the same or are they to be changed? What are the desired goals for both the preceptors and the program? Only when all aspects have been thoroughly reviewed can you proceed.

Several approaches are available to integrate new preceptors into a current system. The methods you originally used to train preceptors, such as workshops, classes, or self-learning can again be used. Assuming a reasonably successful program originally, any will adequately do the job. Reusing your previous approach has the advantage that the format and materials are already established and prepared.

Other alternatives, however, now become possible. The availability of functioning preceptors provides opportunities for training not previously available.

If you have the luxury of adequate time, it may prove helpful to look at having your experienced preceptors assist in training your new ones. A novice can be assigned to a new preceptor with the experienced person assisting the newer one in the skills of precepting. This reinforces and acknowledges experienced preceptors for their expertise, assists the novice preceptor in gaining experience and requisite skills, and still provides an adequate (or better) experience for the novice. In situations where additional preceptors are desired, both the experienced and novice preceptors can then progress to taking their own novices. This approach works extremely well but requires advance planning. In cases where additional fully functioning preceptors are needed immediately, it is more prudent to use one of the original options for training. The ideal is, of course, to combine the two options.

Another option is to incorporate functioning preceptors as instructors or facilitators in classes or workshops. This validates the contributions of current preceptors and gives prospective preceptors firsthand information on the realities of precepting.

Several points must be reiterated when discussing adding preceptors. First, your program is only as good as the preceptors you have. The importance of selecting only those persons suitable as role models cannot be forgotten the second (or third, or fourth, etc.) time around.

Second, precepting requires selected aptitudes and skills. Just as all nurses are not good managers, all nurses are not good preceptors. Don't get excited about a new employee until you've made the appropriate assessments. Furthermore, individuals who act as preceptors must have the desire to precept as well as the ability.

Third, never involve preceptors who do not understand what is required. To do so is unfair. Precepting is rewarding, demanding, frustrating, and time consuming. To involve individuals without an understanding of both the rewards and difficulties is foolish as well. It is, however, always possible (if your system of training allows it financially) to allow individuals to try precepting once and see if they enjoy it. This gives both you and the preceptor the opportunity to opt out if it doesn't work.

Finally, remember that preceptors, as adults, can and should assist in defining their own needs and goals. We, as educators, cannot legislate what individuals ought to learn. If our programs are to be successful, we must assist individuals to diagnose and clarify their own needs and guide them toward meeting the goals they set.

SUMMARY

This chapter has examined improvement and expansion of an existing preceptor program and the new requirements of preceptor recruitment and replacement. Improving or expanding a preceptor program calls for the same careful attention to detail required by the original planning and should be based on sound assessment and program evaluation. This completes our consideration of the development and management of preceptor programs. In Part II we will move on to the development and management of preceptors themselves.

REFERENCE

Knowles, M.S. (1970). *The modern practice of adult education.* New York: Association Press.

Part II

Developing and Managing Preceptors

111

Chapter 9

Assessing Preceptor Needs

This chapter deals with assessing preceptor needs in order to support them in carrying out their responsibilities. Before we begin with that, however, let us review the roles and relationships that make up a preceptor's professional existence.

ROLES AND RELATIONSHIPS

The Preceptor's Role

The planning done by preceptors is on a small scale. The program development outlined in previous chapters is not within the realm of the preceptor but that of the program coordinator. Large-scale planning, system development, budgeting, program planning, interviewing, financial analysis, and the like are rightly under the jurisdiction of the coordinator. The preceptor is responsible for microplanning: deciding which experiences best fit the novice's needs, sequencing experiences so that they build on one another, seeking out learning experiences to meet the novice's needs or goals, and generally planning on a minute-to-minute, hour-to-hour, and day-to-day basis.

Teaching forms a large part of the preceptor's responsibilities. Preceptors must be comfortable with demonstrating new techniques and imparting knowledge in an organized manner on a one-to-one basis. They must be able to take advantage of the situation that comes up unexpectedly and to use questions to facilitate incidental learning. They must be able to build on experiences that the novice already has, proceed from the simple to the complex, and base new information on what is already known.

Preceptors must be social facilitators. They ease the social integration of their novices, including them in unit functions, being sure they are introduced to unfamiliar faces, and generally smoothing the way. The preceptor takes on the responsibility of introducing the novices to staff, accompanying them on rounds or to meetings, and easing them into overall staff membership.

Finally, preceptors are responsible for evaluating others. They must give effective but not overwhelming feedback, be objective yet supportive, and concentrate on behaviors not personalities. They must maintain this relationship despite the fact that they will be evaluating the novice with whom they work. Few if any preceptors have experience in these matters before precepting.

The role relationships that develop between the novice, preceptor, and other members of the health care team are crucial to the fulfillment of these responsibilities. The relationships either enhance or inhibit the aims of the program and the function of the preceptors. Therefore, both preceptors and program coordinators need a clear picture of these relationships.

The Coordinator's Role

As program coordinator you have a unique relationship with the preceptors. As a resource person, you should provide a nonthreatening supportive environment for both preceptors and novices. Your role is that of a facilitator and educator rather than a line supervisor or evaluator. Unless you can establish this type of helping role it will be hard for you to fully develop your preceptors, as they will be uncomfortable coming to you when they experience difficulty. You must be available and willing to respond when they need help. You must respect the difficulties inherent in their role as preceptors and be sensitive to their unspoken as well as spoken needs. You must support their feelings of worth and self-esteem, while helping them to develop in their role.

When comfortable, preceptors will come to you with a variety of concerns. You can help them to give timely and worthwhile feedback and serve as a sounding board for them as they work out solutions, ventilate feelings, and reflect on successes and failures. You can help them to gain perspective on their actions and on the actions of the novices, serve as a mediator to facilitate communication, smooth the difficulties that sometimes arise between head nurses and preceptors, and assist the preceptors in selecting learning experiences that will support desired goals. You can help preceptors assess the novice's progress and write fair and effective evaluations. Above all you must remain accepting and nonjudgmental, supporting them in their role as you assist them to develop their skills.

The Preceptor-Novice Relationship

The relationship that forms between the novice and preceptor is the most crucial link in the chain. A less than satisfactory relationship hinders educational efforts. A variety of factors enter into this relationship, including anxiety, reality shock, confidentiality, empathy, involvement, acceptance, trust, humor, and anxiety.

Anxiety

Anyone accepting a new position is anxious. This normal anxiety is multiplied in the case of novices, unsure of themselves as professionals and fearful about the role and responsibilities to be assumed. While mild anxiety can be helpful to learning, increasing levels interfere in the absorption of new information. Preceptors must be able to recognize the anxiety level of the novice and to keep it at motivating rather than paralyzing levels. Remembering how they felt the first working day after graduation can help preceptors to keep the novice's anxiety in perspective and to plan accordingly.

Reality Shock

Reality shock can be described as the discrepancy between expectations and actual reality, and it hits new graduates hardest (Kramer, 1974). Many believe that all of us go through the stages of reality shock in each job that we accept; however, its effects are the most pronounced in our first professional position, both because we are unprepared for it and because our professional ideals have not yet been impacted by reality.

According to Kramer (1974) and Schmalenberg and Kramer (1979), there are four phases to reality shock. The first phase, often titled the "honeymoon," consists of a time of near euphoria. Everything is wonderful: the job is great, the supervisors understanding and caring, the patients wonderful. The individuals feel they are constantly learning and growing and that their choice of a profession was the best one possible for them.

Gradually, this euphoria disappears and depression sets in. The job suddenly doesn't seem so great, the supervisors turn hard and cynical, the patients are demanding and ungrateful. The hypocrisy of people saying one thing and doing another hits, and life becomes polarized into a "we-they" situation. Life seems to turn into an endless circle consisting of work, eat, sleep, work. Exhausted, apathetic, and generally unhappy, people undergoing reality shock feel dissatisfied with themselves and everyone around them. The views of how nursing ought to be and how it really is seem far apart.

Often this stage proves fatal. Caught in a trap without a visible means of escape, the individual either opts to job hop, looking for the ideal position (which of course doesn't exist); or goes native, abandoning the values learned in school and accepting the prevailing values of the organization; or does a lateral arabesque, returning to school purely for the escape it offers from the real world; or becomes a rutter, simply doing the job because it has to be done; or finally burns out completely and leaves the profession altogether.

If they can force themselves to stick it out long enough, most individuals eventually find themselves in the recovery stage. A new sense of balance prevails and they feel more relaxed and able to cope. Their energy begins to return and life no longer looks so bleak.

The last phase is called *resolution*. It is during this phase that methods for handling some of the conflicts are found and internal conflicts begin to be resolved. The person becomes bicultural, integrating his or her own values into the real world and coming out with a workable, livable compromise between the ideal and reality.

Trust

Throughout their relationship a feeling of trust between the novice and preceptor is essential. This trust extends two ways—the novice must trust the preceptor and the preceptor must grow to trust the novice. Without trust, both novice and preceptor will feel isolated and anxious. Trust can be facilitated by congruence between speech and action and by honesty, consistency, and dependability on the part of both preceptor and novice.

Confidentiality goes along with trust. The novice must be sufficiently comfortable in the relationship to express fears and trepidations and must feel secure that the preceptor will respect confidences. Honesty in the relationship is essential. If a confidence cannot be kept, and at times for various reasons this does occur, the situation should be discussed with the novice before confidences are violated.

Acceptance

Acceptance is also essential to the development of an effective relationship between the preceptor and novice. Nonjudgmental, open-minded attitudes acknowledge differences but still value individuals for their uniqueness. Acceptance does not imply that personal values have to be rejected, but rather acknowledges that each individual has the right to his or her own values and beliefs. This works two ways, since often the novice has as difficult a time as the preceptor accepting the validity of a different value system. Acceptance of the novice as an individual does not mean that offensive behavior is endorsed or accepted, but rather that correction of the behavior still communicates recognition of the person's intrinsic worth. Acceptance implies a willingness to start where the novice is at.

Recognition of a difference in values is often the first and most important step in becoming accepting of others. Massey's book *The People Puzzle* (1979) can help novices and preceptors clarify where their own values lie and stem from and assist them to develop an attitude of acceptance.

Empathy

Empathy on the part of the preceptor is imperative. Empathy is feeling with someone rather than feeling for them. Empathy views an experience through the other person's eyes rather than your own. It is through empathy that subtle or covert needs are recognized. Empathy conveys a willingness to accept the novice's feelings and to work with him or her; to recognize oneself in the novice.

Empathy occurs in two phases. First, one identifies one's similarities with the other person, remembering incidents that evoked similar feelings, for example. Then, feelings of separateness from the other person are identified by defining the differences between their situation and feelings and one's own.

Empathy is not sympathy. In sympathy, self-identity and feeling of separateness are lost. One incorporates the feelings of the person as one's own. In other words, empathy is to feel *with* the people; sympathy to feel *for* them. Sympathy limits one's effectiveness and ability to be objective.

Empathic approaches support mutual problem solving and avoid unnecessary use of authority. Empathy is communicated by involving ourselves in the novice's feelings and thoughts instead of only our own and through physical presence, active listening, and supportive rather than punitive interactions.

Involvement is essential in precepting. The preceptor cannot be an uninvolved bystander but must express an interest in and take an active part in the planning for and development of the novice. The preceptor must care about what happens to the novice. Involvement begins the moment preceptors learn they are to have a novice, intensifies when they first meet and define goals with that novice, and strengthens as they work together to meet goals.

Perspective

A sense of humor is indispensable. This means laughing at ourselves rathe: than at others. Humor serves to relieve stress and tension, strengthen interpersonal relationships, and cement feelings of community. Without the ability to laugh at oneself, precepting would soon become overwhelming.

The Preceptor-Head Nurse Relationship

The preceptor and the head nurse share a unique relationship in the development of the novice. The preceptor, in essence, acts as a surrogate for the head nurse in developing and supporting the novice through the initial stages of professional development. This surrogate role requires mutual respect and the assumption of responsibilities on both sides.

If head nurses cannot see the value of preceptors and the reasons for the program, they will be little support. Preceptors must feel valued and needed for their expertise rather than overloaded. The head nurse must appreciate the difficulties inherent in precepting and support preceptors in their efforts in multiple ways.

In turn preceptors must realize the enormous demands placed on head nurses today and recognize the management role of the head nurse. If preceptors do not recognize the right and responsibility of the head nurse to follow the progress of the novice, they will interpret the head nurse's actions and interest as interference. Mutual respect and understanding is the basis for collaborative problem solving and program support.

Both the head nurse and preceptor have responsibilities for the novice. Even where the novice is hired by nursing administration and is not directly responsible to the head nurse, the head nurse is still responsible for the quality of care that patients receive on the unit. Therefore, head nurses have a direct interest in and responsibility for the novice's practice. It is essential that they be interested in the novice's progress and be supportive of the preceptor. Very often, the head nurse is the preceptor's first line resource for problem-solving assistance, particularly when the coordinator is new or not so well known to the preceptor.

The preceptor must coordinate efforts and goals with the head nurse, particularly if the head nurse still makes assignments. Frequently, minor changes must be made that conflict with normal practice. For example, it may be the practice of the head nurse to assign the same patients for a period of time to the same staff in order to provide as much continuity of care as possible. However, after several days it may be a better learning experience for the novice to switch patients. The head nurse must understand that the preceptor is not requesting this just to be difficult and must respect the preceptor's judgment about where the novice is in the learning situation. Nor should the preceptor be offended if the head nurse corrects the novice or comes to the preceptor about a problem that was observed. The two roles should complement each other, not conflict with each other.

The Preceptor-Staff Relationship

The preceptor serves as a buffer between the novice and other members of the health care team. Until novices are ready to assume the responsibility of interacting with other departments, physicians, or administrative personnel, it will be the preceptors who do so on their behalf, role modeling preferred styles of interaction. Gradually, with coaching from the preceptor the novice assumes this function until the preceptor has bowed out altogether.

The Preceptor-to-Preceptor Relationship

The preceptor-to-preceptor relationship is also important. The goal is an association of peers forming a support group. All preceptors should be considered equal in status; precepting in critical care areas, for example, should not be considered more difficult than precepting on general units. It is important that preceptors build each other up, instead of tearing each other down; upon hearing about each other as well as on a face-to-face basis. Preceptors will hear about other preceptors, especially if novices are rotating among several preceptors. If the things they hear are negative, they should act as impartial listeners if they cannot explain the rationale behind the action. Sometimes it is possible to understand and thus interpret actions for the novice. In other cases, where rationales are not obvious, preceptors should remain nonjudgmental. Concerns about particular preceptors should be referred to the program coordinator.

PRECEPTOR NEEDS

To fulfill these roles preceptors must have a base of knowledge that can be utilized to meet their responsibilities. Preceptors need information about adult learning, teaching techniques, supervising others, evaluating others, communication, time and stress management, and a multitude of other topics if they are to perform effectively. As program coordinator, you must be prepared to help them grow and learn in areas that are unfamiliar.

We discussed general development of the preceptors in Chapters 5, 6, and 8. How do you go about deciding in what areas your preceptors need to develop specific skills?

First, in order to effectively assess needs, you must identify what those needs are. According to Atwood et al. (1971), an educational need is "a need that can be satisfied by means of a learning experience. It is considered to be a lack, deprivation or deficiency that tells one what to do from an educational standpoint." Knowles (1970) identifies an educational need as a gap between the present level of competency and that expected or required.

The purpose of needs assessment, then, is to determine the type and level of specific educational requirements needed to fill the gap. We shall be speaking primarily of preceptor needs here, but the same techniques apply to the assessment of other groups such as novices.

Accurate assessment of the student's learning needs is essential if the process is to be effective. Areas that should be considered are the cognitive, affective, psychomotor, recall, and discrimination skills.

Cognitive skills, as we have noted, relate to knowledge or facts. For example, to write effective nursing care plans, the student must know what a nursing care plan is and what components should be included in the plan. Psychomotor skills are motor skills. In our example above, the student must be able to pick up the pen, put pen to paper, and create symbols that are meaningful to others.

Affective skills relate to attitudes, values, or feelings. These are generally the hardest to teach and take the longest time to integrate into the individual's frame of reference. To complete our example above, the individual must know not only how to write a care plan and what to include, but must see the activity as valuable if the behavior of writing effective nursing care plans is to be continued without the presence of an authority figure to enforce it.

Recall refers to the ability to retain information and return it to the conscious mind for use when it is needed. The information may refer to any of the areas mentioned above: cognitive, affective, or psychomotor. It is impossible for any of us to retain all the information we possess on a conscious level. We would soon become overloaded and burn out. However, the ability to recall the information is essential if it is to be available when needed. This means that the material must be learned thoroughly enough that it is filed completely, without gaps that will prohibit effective recall and use later.

Discrimination is the final area of assessment. To really understand, the learner must be able to distinguish small differences between instances. Similarly, the learner must be able to generalize, to see how things are similar in overall ways. Frequently, discrimination and generalization are left out of objectives when actually it is these skills that are the most important to be learned.

Who Does the Assessment?

Needs assessment may be carried out either by the learner or others. At least some element of self-diagnosis is essential for adult learners. Most adults are aware, at least to some extent, of their needs, and we have noted that adults learn best in situations where they have played at least a part in determining what is to be learned.

Knowles (1970) identifies three phases in self-assessment: constructing a competency model or the characteristics needed for ideal performance, defining the present level of competency, and measuring the gaps between the desired and present levels of competency.

How Is Assessment Done?

Needs can be defined by three methods. The individuals themselves can be asked what they need; persons in helping roles can be asked what is needed; or experts can be asked what is needed.

Self assessment formats provide ways for adults to identify their own performance, and compare it to others or a standard. One of the easiest ways to do this is with a self assessment form. Knowledge, skills, and attitudes necessary for success are identified and placed on the form. Adults then rate themselves, and identify areas for further learning. Priorities can be described as a part of the assessment, if that is desired. Remember that any form you develop should be based on the values and competencies desired for your particular program. (The appendix includes several examples of preceptor self assessment forms.)

Utilizing self diagnosis obligates one to base content on the expressed needs. Educators must be prepared to be flexible; they must incorporate the desires of their learners into their plans. If they are unwilling or unable to do so, learners should not be asked to participate in any type of assessment. Assessing needs establishes an unwritten contract between learner and teacher, implying that the needs identified will be met, at least partially.

Self assessment identifies felt needs. However, "unfelt" or observed needs may also need to be addressed.

Persons in adjacent or helping roles can be asked to define such unfelt needs. Head nurses, program coordinators, past preceptors, administrators, or novices can be queried on needs and competencies of preceptors and their information pooled to form a composite picture of needs. In addition, new trends, program revisions, or management suggestions may need to be incorporated into educational planning.

Many of these aspects can be covered by asking experts. Experts include not only persons who have run preceptor programs but also the literature, professional norms and trends, and the like. In all likelihood, at least some component of the experts' opinion will be included, but be careful to reflect the desires of your own program rather than those of the experts.

A multiplicity of means can be used to directly obtain information from each of these and other sources. Bell (1978) identifies 18 different techniques, and numerous other authors have discussed additional ones. Exhibit 9-1 provides a summary of assessment techniques. Common methods of needs assessment include buzz groups, checklists, interviews, tests, questionnaires, advisory groups, activity analyses, observations, chart audits, performance appraisals, and suggestion boxes.

Buzz groups may be conducted in several ways. The group may be divided into small groups (from three to six persons) and given five to ten minutes to discuss what they would like more information on. A spokesperson is appointed and suggestions are pooled. This may be helpful if group members are unfamiliar with one another as it builds in interaction and individual contributions. Alternatively, a pyramid scheme can be used, where two persons discuss needs and come up with a mutual consensus. Two dyads then join to form a group of four and renegotiate a consensus. That group then joins with another group of four and the process is repeated. This facilitates the development of one set of mutually agreed upon needs, but loses the special needs one individual might have.

Checklists are a common means of needs assessment, as they are easy to develop and analyze. A series of items are listed and perceived areas of need are indicated by checking or circling. As variations on checklists, items may be rated ("great need," "moderate need," "little or no need") or ranked (top five

Exhibit 9-1 Summary of Needs Assessment Techniques

Technique	Suitable for Assessing			Useful For			Use For Input From				Use for Input About			
	Structure	Performance	Knowledge	Individual	Small Group	Large Group	Novice	Preceptors	Other Key People	Others	Novices	Preceptors	Program	Trends
Advisory Groups	X	X	X			X	?	?	X					
Literature Review	X		X	X	X					X				X
Institution Reports	X	X	X		X					X				v
Checklists	X	X	X	X	X	X	X	X	X		X	X	X	?
Personal Interview	X	X	X	X	X		X	X	X		X	X	X	X
Re-diagnosis			X	X	X	X	X	X			X	X		
Written Survey	X	X	X	X	X	?	X	X	X		X	X	X	X
Tests			X	X	X	X	X	X			X	X	?	
Skill Inventories		X	X	X	X	X	X	X			X	X		
Buzz Groups	X	X	?		X	X	X	X	X		X	X	X	?
Questionnaires	X	X	?		X	X	X	X	X		X	X	X	X
Activity Analysis		X	X		X	X	X	X	X		X	X	X	
Observations		X	?	X	X		X	X	X		X	X	X	?
Chart Audits		X	X	X	X	X	X			X	X	?		
Performance Appraisals		X		X	X	X		X	X		X	X		

? = May have application in some circumstances

items = highest need). Appendix K contains an example of a checklist for needs assessment.

Interviews may be done either with groups or individuals. If the group is small enough, it is sometimes useful to use a matrix format where people jot down or discuss what they would like to learn. The matrix is composed of names vertically and interest areas horizontally (see Exhibit 9-2); each person adds additional areas he or she would like covered during the discussion or in response to the assessor's questions.

Tests are also an option. Such objective measures give clear-cut indications of gaps between expected and actual knowledge. Care must be taken when constructing test items that they truly reflect what is necessary knowledge and that the effect of non-knowledge-related factors, such as anxiety, are taken into account when analyzing results.

Exhibit 9-2 Matrix Needs Assessment Format

	Performance Evaluation	Teaching Techniques	Communication	Time Management	Adult Development
CJ	X			X	
MJ	X		X	X	
SK	X	X	X		X
NB	X	X		X	X
	4	2	2	3	2

Questionnaires are undoubtedly one of the most popular ways to assess needs. Before they are circulated widely, they should be piloted with a small group to be sure questions are clear and easy to tabulate. Open-ended or projective questions, those that ask respondents how they would act or feel in a given situation, often elicit helpful information. An analysis of answers to questions such as "If you and a novice disagreed about patient priorities, what would you do?" or "If you were to have a new novice tomorrow, what questions would you ask him or her?" can help to diagnose where gaps are between desired and actual performance.

Advisory committees are another method of needs assessment. If groups are large, an advisory group may be the only way to obtain representative information from group members. Key people from groups other than the target group can be included and representatives can solicit input from those they represent.

Activity analysis examines the major tasks, knowledge, and attitudes required of the target group and identifies necessary competencies. This is often the first step in developing a competency-based model and may form the basis for self-assessment tools.

Focus observations assist in determining needs. Such methods include direct observation of individual or group performance. These observations are often helpful in identifying unfelt needs but they may be unduly influenced by the observer's unrecognized biases.

Formal or informal chart audits or reviews of performance appraisals can reveal needs that may go unrecognized by group members. Such an analysis can point up areas of deficiency or gaps that relate directly to learning needs.

Suggestion boxes provide an anonymous way to gather information. If locations are carefully selected, they also enable the writer to deposit an entry at the time when the need is first perceived or identified. This helps to capture needs that might otherwise be missed.

Having reviewed alternatives, you must now make your choices and do the actual assessment. Exhibit 9-3 can help you outline your plan.

Analyzing the Data

Once data have been gathered, they must be analyzed. This analysis usually follows the steps of review, classification, interpretation, and evaluation of the data.

First, needs should be reviewed to be sure that information is complete and easily understood. If it is not, further discussion with the parties involved may be necessary before analysis continues.

Next, the data must be classified. There are a number of ways in which to do this. One suggestion would be to review the information and sort out learning needs from other types of needs. Often additional needs, such as those for equipment or personnel, become entwined with learning needs as they are assessed. It is a good idea to set these aside for the moment if interruptions for clarification would prove disruptive.

Exhibit 9-3 Learning Needs Assessment Plan

Purpose of assessment:

What do I want to discover?

Who will develop the tool or do the assessment?

Who will be assessed?

Using what format?

When will it be done?

You will need to screen for duplication and to group items that naturally seem to go together. For example, you may see individual contributions having to do with giving criticism, preparing time guidelines for evaluations, and making evaluations. These may be grouped under one broader umbrella of evaluations.

As you interpret and evaluate the data, several questions should be kept in mind. Are there other programs of offerings that will meet this need? Nothing says that your program must meet each and every individual need; wise use of the resources around you can save time, money, and energy.

Does this need relate directly to the program and is it necessary? Your resources are limited; therefore address those needs that relate directly and necessarily to the function of the program first. There may or may not be time and resources to address the others.

Is it feasible to meet this need? Is there sufficient interest and need to warrant the time and expense involved? Some items may also have to be excluded as they conflict with program or institutional goals or philosophies: an expressed desire by preceptors for information on formal classroom instruction techniques, for example, may conflict with the philosophy of one-to-one hands-on instruction; or a desire for information on evaluation may be impractical in a facility that does not expect evaluations of its preceptors.

Set priorities. Some needs will obviously be more important than others or may need to precede others to make sense. If many seem to be equally important, sequencing is not an issue, and priorities were not included in your original assessment, consider asking those who participated in the assessment to rank the needs identified in order of importance to them. Be careful not to determine priorities solely on the respondents' replies; organizational or program factors often take precedence.

Finally, translate the remaining needs into learning objectives. From those objectives a program can be developed that focuses, as adult education should, on the identified needs of the program participants.

SUMMARY

This chapter has discussed assessment of needs in order to aid preceptors in fulfilling their responsibilities. The remaining chapters will offer specific information on topics identified as being most needed by preceptors. Chapter 10 begins with adult learning.

REFERENCES

Atwood, H., et al. (1971). Concept of need: An analysis for adult education. *Adult Leadership*, *19*(1), 212. Cited in D.F. Bell. (1978). Assessing educational needs: Advantages and disadvantages of eighteen techniques. *Nurse Educator*, *3*(5), 15–21.

Knowles, M.S. (1970). *The modern practice of adult education*. New York: Association Press.

Kramer, M. (1974). *Reality shock: Why nurses leave nursing*. St. Louis: Mosby.

Massey, M. (1979). *The people puzzle: Understanding yourself and others*. Reston, VA: Reston Publishing.

Schmalenberg, C., & Kramer, M. (1979) *Coping with reality shock: The voices of experience*. Wakefield, MA: Nursing Resources.

Chapter 10

Principles of Adult Education

This chapter will deal with the subject of adults and how they learn. For many, the idea that adults learn differently from children will be a new and perhaps startling one. Conditioned to believe that both children and adults learn in similar manners, we have difficulty accepting the fact that the ways in which we learned to learn as children are not the only options. Yet when we examine the ways in which we as adults incorporate new information, we find them quite different from those used by children.

Webster (1967) defines *adult* as one who is "fully developed and mature; grown-up." Knowles (1970) defines the adult as one who has come to see himself as self-directing, preferring this psychological description as more accurate than either the legal or physiological definitions.

Learning, as defined by McLagan (1978), is:

> a change in knowledge, behavior, attitudes/values/priorities or creativity that can result when learners interact with information. It occurs to the extent that learners are motivated to change, and is applied in the real world to the extent that they take successful steps to integrate that learning into the real world situation. (p. 1)

Until the twentieth century, it was assumed that adults learn in exactly the same manner that children do. Between World War I and World War II, investigators confirmed that there were indeed differences in the ways in which adults and children learn. This knowledge has gradually evolved into the theory of adult learning we now accept. The modern theories of adult learning (and this chapter) owe a great deal to Malcolm Knowles (1970), who did much of the synthesis of abstract ideas into a workable theory and who coined the word *andragogy* to describe adult learning. (*Pedagogy* is the art and science of teaching children.)

CHARACTERISTICS OF ADULTS AS LEARNERS

What distinguishes the adult as a learner from the child? First, adults have an independent self-concept. They are self-directed, while children are other-directed. Children move from total dependence on others to a slowly developed independence, but always rely on parents, teachers, or peers for direction and guidance. Adults, by contrast, are guided by their own knowledge and beliefs and are resentful and resistant when not allowed to set their own direction and abide by their own counsel.

Adults have a broad experiential base. Their experiences provide an extensive background on which to base and relate new information and yield a wealth of information to share with others. In addition, adults define themselves through their experiences. Their experiences provide validation and substantiation for who they are as human beings. Furthermore, adults organize their experiences in unique ways; each person individualizes his or her experiences and interprets similar experiences differently. Children, by contrast, lack a broad background of experience on which to base new learning and tend to define experiences as something that happens to them, rather than as something in which they participate.

Adults and children also differ in their readiness to learn. Adults' readiness to learn is determined by their developmental stage and the resultant tasks to be accomplished. Andragogy maintains that adults learn because of the requirements of their roles as husbands and wives, mothers and fathers, nurses, committee chairpeople, skiers, and the like. Pedagogy, on the other hand, assumes that children are ready to learn as a result of their biological age and academic level.

Adults require immediacy of application for optimal learning. Most of children's learning requires postponed application—the child learns in grade school what will be needed in high school several years later. Adults, on the other hand, need to see an application for the learning at the time it occurs. The sooner the material is to be applied, the greater the stimulus to learn. Adults simply aren't interested in learning things they might need "one day."

Adults have a problem-centered orientation. They are interested in learning information that will help them to cope with their developmental tasks, their social roles, and everyday life. If an adult feels that the material being presented can help solve current problems or more satisfactorily fulfill a social role, learning will be enhanced.

Adults have a changing physiological state. As we grow older, we face mental, emotional, and biological changes. It becomes more difficult to take information in because hearing or visual losses take their toll. Our mobility decreases and with it some of our options for information gathering. These changes may provoke learning—how to walk with a cane to increase our mobility, for example—but in other cases learning is inhibited.

From these characteristics, a pattern of the adult as a learner begins to emerge. The adult is a self-directed, practical, problem-solving individual who relies on past experiences to aid learning and who seeks immediate application of learning. Learning needs evolve from and center on social roles and developmental tasks. The pedagogical learner, on the other hand, is dependent, relies little on past experience, is subject-centered, plans on postponed application, and is dependent on biological age and social pressures to determine readiness for learning.

FACTORS AFFECTING ADULT LEARNING

Many factors affect the adult learner. These help to determine the adult's readiness to absorb and synthesize new information and dictate the motivation for doing so.

Self-Concept

First is the individual adult's self-concept. Society defines the role of children as that of learners. Adults, on the other hand, define themselves (and are defined by others) as producers or doers, not learners. Adults are internally directed with well-developed self-concepts. They are independent and need not define themselves as children do by input from others. Adults need to have respect, to make their own decisions, and to be seen as unique persons.

At the same time, most adults do not recognize themselves as learners at all. Despite research which shows that most adults are active self-directed learners— Moran (1977), for example, found that nurses averaged 469 hours per year of independent study—many individuals think of themselves as the old dog that can't be taught new tricks. When faced with the "student" role, many adults find themselves, by their own definition, unable to cope.

Because of the demands of their profession, nurses are probably more comfortable with the learner role than many other adults. Clark and Dickson (1976), in a study on self-directed versus other-directed continuing education, found that all the nurses in their study participated to some extent in continuing education activities, that the majority of nurses had a positive attitude toward continued learning, and that they participated more in self-directed than other-directed activities.

Environment

The environment has a definite effect on the adult learner. Adults are accustomed to a degree of autonomy in their physical climates and resent being made to feel uncomfortable. An environment that provides comfortable seating, adequate ventilation and warmth, where participants are able to see and hear satisfactorily, where breaks are planned periodically, and where restroom facilities are available will enhance learning.

Adults are also accustomed to some freedom in their psychological climate and resent being "held" in an uncomfortable setting. Open, nonauthoritarian atmospheres stimulate adult learner involvement, initiative, and creativity, and encourage self-confidence, originality, and independence. All of these enhance learning. Adults need to feel adequate, competent, and secure. Environments where the participants feel talked down to, embarrassed, threatened, or intimidated block learning.

Age

Mental decline is a frequent concern for those who will teach adults. A common myth is that adults decline in learning abilities as they grow older. In fact, learning ability does not decline with age. Brain cells remain active until senility. Evidence suggests that older persons decline only in areas that require quick reactions and decisions (Stein, 1971). It is generally recognized, however, that adult learners are more prone to rigid thinking than children, as preconceptions and previously learned concepts and ways of doing things limit unique interpretations of data and creative solutions to problems. In addition, learning may take longer for the adult as previous ways of doing things must sometimes be unlearned before new information can be incorporated.

Some physical conditions, however, do decline with age. Vision becomes dimmer, hearing becomes less acute, muscles become stiffer. Memory may become less acute. Energy levels and reserves decline. In general, aging produces a diminishing ability to adapt to physical and psychological stress (Granick & Patterson, 1971). This has obvious implications for adult educators who want to maintain an optimal learning environment, as they must adjust the environment to accommodate these deficiencies.

Life experiences are obviously major determinants for adult learners. Adults define and validate themselves by their past experiences and judge their own and others' experiences in light of both current and traditional definitions of cultural, social, religious, and institutional correctness. They recognize their own experiences as valuable and want others to do the same. New experiences are viewed within the framework of past ones. This has significance for the educator, who will find each learner has unique experiences, even if settings are identical, as each individual categorizes, integrates, and views experiences differently.

The adult's developmental stage affects the ability and motivation to learn. Differences in maturation, task accomplishments, and constitutional capacity influence both what is learned and the rate of that learning. Adults learn, in part, because they feel the need to develop knowledge or competency in the tasks that life gives them. For example, individuals have little motivation or interest in learning parenting skills until they become parents and then this becomes a major focus. Table 10-1 presents two differing views on the developmental tasks of adults, those of Havighurst and Orr (1956) and Sheehy (1976).

Demands on one's time result from the requirements of developmental tasks. Educational needs often must take a back seat for adults as they struggle to meet the day-to-day claims of family, job, community, and religion.

Motivation

Motivation is a prerequisite for optimal learning. Learning is facilitated when individuals see the relationship between what is being learned and their personal needs, problems, or goals. Adults are also interested in learning for its own sake, but they want learning to help them solve the problems they are currently facing.

Motivation can be either internal ("I want to learn this because I am interested in it and need more information") or external ("If you don't learn this you will lose your job "). Internal motivations are stronger than external motivations.

Table 10-1 Development during Adult Years

Havighurst and Orr	Sheehy

Early adulthood (18 to 30)
    Selecting a mate
    Starting and raising a family
    Selecting an occupation
	Pulling up roots (18 to 20)
	    Leaving home
	    Locating self in peer group, occupation,
	      and viewpoints

Middle age (30 to 55)
    Achieving recognition in community
    Maintaining a standard of living
    Adjusting to physiological changes
    Relating to one's spouse as a person
	Trying twenties (20 to 30)
	    Relating with external situations
	
	 Catch-30 (30 to 35)
	    Tearing up what was done in 20s
	    Having new energies

Later maturity (55 and over)
    Adjusting to physical limitations
    Adjusting to retirement and death of
      spouse
    Meeting community obligations
	Deadline decade (35 to 45)
	    Intense concentration on advancement
	
	 Renewal or resignation (45 to 50)
	    Regaining equilibrium
	    Emphasis on friends and privacy

From *The Process of Staff Development: Components for Change* (2nd ed.) (p. 79), by H. Tobin, P. Yoder Wise, and P. Hull, 1979, St. Louis: C.V. Mosby. Copyright 1979 by C.V. Mosby. Reprinted by permission.

McClusky's concept of margin can help us to understand the motivation of adults (Gessner, 1979).

The concept of margin involves load, power, and margin. *Power* is the sum of the individual's resources. These include physical, psychological, social, cultural, spiritual, cognitive, and economic traits and are the assets the individual uses to deal with load. *Load* refers to the demands placed on the individual. The demands may be familial, religious, societal, economic, or the like and include the expectations imposed on oneself by both others and self.

> If the person's responsibilities (load) are equal to or greater than his capabilities (power), the individual has no margin and is unable to function effectively. However, when power is greater than load, the person has developed a surplus of power, hence he has margin. Having margin allows the person to undertake new challenges or deal with stresses. (Gessner, 1979, p. 40)

Motivations to learn vary greatly among individuals. Clark and Dickson (1976), concurring with earlier researchers, found that the nurses in their study had seven basic motivations for continued learning: meeting occupational, professional, or societal goals; learning; sociability; relief from boredom and frustration; and interaction with others.

Education and Learning Style

Education is a factor in the desire to pursue continued learning. One's reading level and comfort level with pursuing the type of learning offered are sure to affect the diligence with which one pursues further education. Learning style will also help or hinder; we are more likely to pursue types of education that fit the styles of learning we prefer.

Kolb's tool for assessing learning styles provides a beginning point for examining preferences. Kolb (1979a) describes four modes of learning: concrete experience, reflective observation, abstract conceptualization, and active experimentation. Shaw and Phillips (1982) have further developed his work.

It must be stressed that none of these styles is inherently good or bad. Lingering in one phase is a reflection of personal preference and past experiences. "The key to effective learning is being competent in each mode when it is appropriate" (Kolb, Rubin, & McIntyre, 1974).

Each of us uses all of the styles. The process of learning forms a cycle, with each of us progressing through all stages but "lingering at those we most prefer" (Shaw & Phillips, 1982).

The cycle progresses from concrete experience, which provides the raw data from observation, experience, or feelings, to observation and reflection. In this phase the learner reflects on individual experiences and reactions from the first stage. Next, generalizations are formed during the abstract conceptualization phase, and finally new hypotheses are formed that generate and are tested in new concrete experiences.

Learners who prefer concrete experience are those who rely heavily on past experiences to help them put new information into perspective. They rely on experience to help them categorize and synthesize new information, and they continue to try out new approaches based on past successes and failures. These learners prefer personal involvement and generally find the theoretical approaches less than helpful. They tend to be empathetic and people oriented and prefer less authoritarian learning situations. They enjoy discussion groups and find specific examples in which they can become personally involved helpful.

Reflective observers prefer observation of what is happening around them to personal involvement. Synthesis and learning of new information are based on logical analysis of what they have heard or seen. These learners are generally introverts, prefer impersonal learning situations such as lectures, and are often seen as passive.

Abstract conceptualizers are those who are able to form abstract theories and concepts about what is happening to them. They are logical and analytical learners and rely on formation of the conceptual framework within which to integrate new learning. They prefer impersonal learning situations, dislike self-learning types of activities, and prefer receiving direction in their learning from authority figures.

Active experimenters are those learners who have an active, involved approach to learning. Generally extroverts, they prefer personal involvement and participatory activities and dislike authority-directed or passive learning situations.

Because we do not fall strictly into one category, Kolb's research has been extended, and combinations, more descriptive of individual styles, have been identified. These styles are divergers, assimilators, convergers, and accommodators. (See Figure 10-1.)

Divergers blend concrete experience and reflective observation. They are creative, imaginative individuals who excel in developing a myriad of alternatives from a single situation or piece of information. These are the idea people, the ones who are best at generating new alternatives and ways of looking at things. True-false or multiple-choice questions drive these learners crazy—they just don't see that one answer can be the only correct one. They much prefer discussion groups or brainstorming sessions where there is opportunity for personal involvement. These people-oriented individuals tend to gravitate toward liberal arts or humanities professions: counseling, personnel management, consulting, and the like.

On the other hand, assimilators, the combination of reflective observers and abstract conceptualizators, are those who can take diverse bits of information

Figure 10-1 Kolb's Cognitive Learning Model

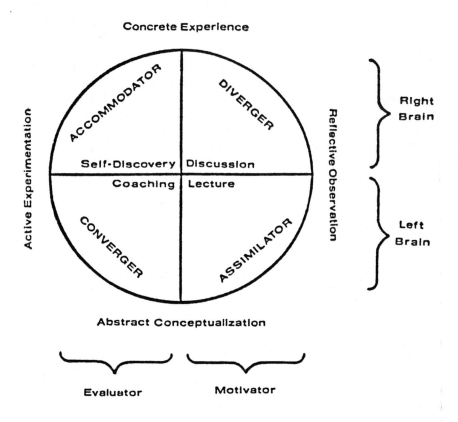

From *Kolb's Cognitive Learning Model* by M. Shaw and S. Phillips. Paper presented at the meeting of the American Society of Health Education and Training, April 16, 1982.

and form them into patterns. They are uniquely able to synthesize new information into theoretical models. Assimilators prefer things to people and occasionally have difficulty in accommodating what actually is rather than what
should be. Assimilators like lectures and are more comfortable in impersonal
learning situations. These individuals tend to gravitate toward the basic sciences
or research and development types of positions.

Convergers, who combine abstract conceptualization and active experimentation, excel in situations where there is one right answer. They are at their
strongest when practically applying ideas, but may have difficulty in accepting
the fact that there is more than one right way to approach a problem. They prefer
impersonal, unemotional situations, and tend to congregate in the physical sci-

ences or engineering. A significant number of nurses fall into this category (Kolb, 1976b).

Accommodators combine concrete experience and active experimentation. These are the "doers," carrying out plans generated by the other three styles. They are the trial-and-error learners and may be less than efficient in their learning patterns. These are the individuals who prefer to throw out the theory when it doesn't match with the reality: "Just stick with the facts"; "Let's do it, not just talk about it." Often found in business, sales, or marketing, these individuals are sometimes seen as pushy by persons with differing styles.

Of what use is all this information? If we know the learning styles of those we seek to instruct, our teaching can be tailored to meet the ways in which those individuals best learn. This saves us both time and frustration and meets the learner's needs instead of our own.

LEARNING PRINCIPLES

When one examines the information in this chapter so far, several basic principles of learning become apparent. The most important of these have to do with reinforcement, readiness to learn, goals and motivations, and learning environments.

Reinforcement

Reinforcement, in learning, is "any event following a response that strengthens it or that increases the probability of the response occurring again" (McNeil & Rubin, 1977). Two types of reinforcement exist: positive and negative. In positive reinforcement a rewarding stimulus is presented after the response to strengthen it. In negative reinforcement, a response is strengthened by the removal of an unpleasant stimulus.

We know from research on learning that behaviors that are reinforced are more likely to recur. Positive reinforcement is a strong motivation to learning, and it is enhanced if it takes place immediately after a successful attempt. For example, if praise is given just after a shoulder sling is correctly applied, repetition of the correct application is more likely to occur than if no praise or criticism is given.

The reverse, however, is not true. Threat and punishment are not, psychologically, the reverse of reward. The threat of punishment does not help the learner to find and fix incorrect responses, and negative reinforcement is generally inappropriate for adult learners.

The greatest reinforcer is a sense of self-satisfaction by the learner. False praise (or reinforcement) by others is of little use. Adults receive little satisfaction in fooling themselves, and internal rewards are far more important than external ones.

Readiness

The participant's readiness to learn affects the quality and quantity of learning. Postponement of learning beyond readiness wastes valuable and often unsuspected learning opportunities, thereby reducing the amount of material that can be mastered in a given period (Conley, 1973). Psychological and physiological maturity, the perception of significance regarding the material or skills to be learned, and freedom from threat are factors determining readiness to learn. Also important are external demands on the individual, the ability to learn in relationship to what is already known, and the perception that the material to be taught can be learned.

The individual's physiological and psychological maturity are important factors. Maturity in adults is for the most part determined by the demands of social roles. We seek information on teaching when we assume a role that demands that we teach; we seek information on hearing aids when it becomes obvious to us that our physiological state demands it. Until that time we resist learning what appears to us to be irrelevant.

Extensive demands on us by others are the norm for modern adults. We must continually balance the demands of family, work, religion, and leisure. Our lives are complex, and are becoming ever more so. Our choices broaden daily, forcing us to select those activities that mean the most to us. An omnipresent statement heard by educators is "I don't have time to attend x." In reality, it is not that we don't have time but that we don't have a current need for the information or perceive it as important and are therefore not yet ready to learn it.

Freedom from threat is an important determinant for our readiness to learn. The possibility of physical or psychological harm inhibits learning. In threatening situations we prepare to fight or flee, not to learn. In tense or traumatic situations, individuals may need frequent repetition of what is to be learned or repeated successful experiences before learning occurs. Adults must feel physically and psychologically comfortable for optimal learning to occur.

Previously learned skills or capabilities play an important part in determining subsequent learning. When new materials build on what has been previously acquired, learners are able to put new information into perspective and see its relation to the whole. For example, if a new monitoring system is similar in configuration to the old one, the learner can compare and contrast the differences mentally and learning is enhanced. If the learner has never before seen a monitor, learning starts at another level and requires additional time.

Goals and Feedback

The perception that we can learn what is to be taught is essential to mastery. Unless we truly believe that we are teachable, our convictions will block our learning. Convincing ourselves may require that we set small goals for ourselves (or for our learners) and that we receive (or give) positive feedback after each small success.

The adult's goals and motivations play a part in determining learning ability. Adults learn best that which they participate in selecting and planning themselves. Learners progress only as far as they have set their own goals. New demands and opportunities increase motivation as learners meet original goals and surpass them. Setting obtainable goals at small intervals so that success is achieved often will help learners to feel stimulated and rewarded. Learning activities must relate to the goals and motivations of the learners if they are to be successful.

Assessment

At least some element of self-diagnosis is essential for adult learners. The individual in question must determine at least in part what their own learning needs are. Self-diagnosis involves the adult looking at self-performance, comparing it with that of others (or an accepted and mutually agreed on standard), and judging where particular strengths and weaknesses lie. Such activities as role playing, simulations, skill practice opportunities, observation, and self-rating scales may be useful in assisting adults to diagnose their own needs. Chapter 8 more thoroughly covers methods of self-assessment for the learner.

Numerous strategies are available to assist in identifying the learning needs of others. Observation of performance includes all types of direct observation of the learner's interaction with others. This may involve direct supervision of the learner; attendance at shift-to-shift report; review of assessments, nursing care plans, and notes; observation of clinical and technical tasks; and making patient rounds to identify, with the learner, learning needs.

Communication techniques include listening to the novices' or preceptors' own assessment of their learning needs; comparing current performance with written standards or expectations; skills lists; learning contracts; performance appraisals; active listening; and informal conferences. Here again, refer to Chapter 8 for a more thorough discussion of learner assessments.

SUMMARY

Adult learners are self-directed and self-disciplined. They learn best when involved in the assessment and planning to meet their identified needs and are affected by a broad variety of both internal and external factors. In the next chapter we shall direct our attention to the next logical step, turning from learning principles and needs of the adult learner to the teaching techniques best suited to them.

REFERENCES

Clark, K.M., & Dickson, G. (1976). Self-directed and other-directed continuing education: A study of nurses' participation. *Journal of Continuing Education in Nursing*, 7(4), 16–24.

Conley, V. (1973). *Curriculum and instruction in nursing*. Boston: Little, Brown.

Gessner, B.A. (1979). McClusky's concept of margin. *Journal of Continuing Education in Nursing*, 10(2), 39–44.

Granick, S., & Patterson, R. (1971). *Human aging II: An eleven year follow-up*. (DHEW Publication No. HSM 71-9037). Washington, D.C.: U.S. Government Printing Office. In H.C. Moidel, E.C. Giblin, & B.M. Wagner (Eds.). (1976). *Nursing care of the patient with medical-surgical disorders* (2nd ed.). New York: McGraw-Hill.

Havighurst, R.J., & Orr, B. (1956). *Adult education and adult needs*. Chicago: Center for the Study of Liberal Education for Adults.

Knowles, M.S. (1970). *The modern practice of adult education*. New York: Association Press.

Kolb, D.A. (1976a). *Learning style inventory: Self scoring test and interpretation booklet*. Boston: McBer and Company.

Kolb, D.A. (1976b). *Learning style inventory: Technical manual*. Boston: McBer and Company.

Kolb, D.A., Rubin, I., & McIntyre, J. (1974a). *Organizational psychology: A book of readings* (2nd ed.). Englewood Cliffs, NJ: Prentice-Hall.

Kolb, D.A., Rubin, I., & McIntyre, J. (1974b). *Organizational psychology: An experiential approach*. Englewood Cliffs, NJ: Prentice-Hall.

McLagan, P.A. (1978). *Helping others learn: Designing programs for adults*. Reading, MA: Addison-Wesley.

McNeil, E.B., & Rubin, Z. (1977). *The psychology of being human* (2nd ed.). San Francisco: Canfield Press.

Moran, V. (1977). Study of comparison of independent learning activities vs. attendance at staff development by staff nurses. *Journal of Continuing Education in Nursing*, 8(3), 14–21.

Shaw, M., & Phillips, S. (1982, April 16). *Kolb's cognitive learning model*. Paper presented at the meeting of the American Society of Health Education and Training. Seattle, Wa.

Sheehy, G. (1976). *Passages: Predictable crises of adult life*. New York: Dutton.

Stein, L.S. (1971). The individual curriculum and nursing leadership. *Journal of Continuing Education in Nursing*, 2(6), 7–13.

Webster's seventh new collegiate dictionary. (1967). Springfield, MA: G. & C. Merriam.

Chapter 11

Effective Teaching

In the last chapter we discussed the principles of adult learning. We now turn our attention to the next logical step—putting those principles into action. This chapter discusses effectively teaching others.

Stop for just a moment and think about the best teacher you've had or one you particularly liked. What made them so effective or enjoyable? Jot some of your thoughts down.

Now think of the worst teacher you've had. What made him or her so much worse? When you examine the behaviors, certain characteristics stand out as being either present or absent. What makes teaching successful, and what are the characteristics of effective teachers?

CHARACTERISTICS OF EFFECTIVE TEACHERS

First, effective teachers are knowledgeable. They are accurate, up-to-date, and practical. Experts in their subject matter, they aren't afraid to divert their attention to answer questions or explore an area of interest to their students. They are well read within their subject, familiar with the specialized aspects of its practice, and comfortable with the practical aspects as well as the theoretical.

Effective teachers are organized. Their content presentation is sequential and follows a logical progression. Presentations are planned and their structure ordered. Key points are identified. They respect time and stick to the allotted time frames.

Effective teachers are stimulating. They both convey knowledge and make it exciting. They use their voices, body movements, and humor to exhibit enjoyment of the subject matter and of teaching. They are enthusiastic.

Effective teachers are competent. They are at ease with the practical skills and techniques of their profession and aren't fazed by the unexpected. They are adept at problem identification, assessment, and intervention and skillful in technical tasks.

Effective teachers provide role models, an ideal for us to strive toward. They are self-confident, but not arrogant, and are not afraid to acknowledge that they don't know it all. They take responsibility for their actions and maintain high professional standards. They respect others, knowing that each of us has individual and unique strengths and weaknesses.

Effective teachers are able to supervise others. They provide coaching and feedback. They are available to their students and are not afraid to provide needed correction as well as praise and encouragement.

Many of the characteristics mentioned above will stand out as being either present in your best teachers or missing in your worst teachers. Luckily, not all characteristics must be inborn for an individual to become an effective teacher. Most teaching skills can be learned.

THE TEACHING PROCESS

According to Knowles (1970), teaching is the process of helping another person to learn. A teacher is unable to really teach in the sense of *making* another person learn, but instead serves as a catalyst for the learner, coinquiring, supplying resources, and facilitating the transaction. Conley states that teaching "refers primarily to the human interaction between teacher and student" (Conley, 1973, p. 391).

In essence the teaching process is similar to the nursing process. One must assess and diagnose what the student's learning needs and preferred ways of learning are, plan to meet the diagnosed needs, implement the plan, and evaluate to be sure the desired outcomes have been met. As in the nursing process, the effort should be a joint one between instructor and student, and the teacher should serve as a facilitator and motivator for the student. Exhibit 11-1 shows this process schematically.

Dealing as we are with adults, the process must be a joint endeavor between student and teacher. We cannot decide what others must learn. We can help them to see a need for the material and assist them in deciding the best way to pursue the desired knowledge, but only the learner can decide that the material is of significant value to warrant the investment of time and energy. Since adults have a variety of demands on their time, the material must meet a perceived need if it is to be effectively "taught." The only way to be sure that the material will fill that need is to involve the learner in the planning process.

Assessing Needs and Planning

Accurate assessment of the student's learning needs is essential if the process is to be effective. Areas that should be considered are the cognitive, affective, psychomotor, recall, and discrimination skills, discussed in Chapter 10.

Exhibit 11-1 The Teaching Process

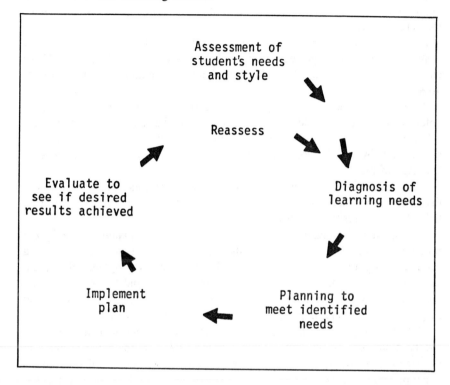

After assessing the needs of students and diagnosing specific areas of need, the next step is planning to meet those needs. Why must you plan for instruction? You plan to ensure your own comfort. It is disconcerting, to say the least, to find yourself in the position of having to teach material with which you are not familiar or where you have not had a chance, even if briefly, to think through how you will present the material or concepts.

Planning also ensures that there is adequate time for the material to be covered, facilitates organization and prioritization, ensures that needed supplies or equipment can be gathered, keeps you centered on the material at hand, permits incorporation of time for review of content when that is necessary, allows you to choose the best format for presentation of the material, decreases time spent on trial-and-error approaches, and makes better use of everyone's time. The key to successful teaching is effective planning.

This does not necessarily mean that a great deal of time must be spent in planning. When precepting, it is common to have procedures or activities come up unexpectedly. One need not plan every sentence. But planning must occur, even if it is only to run quickly through the procedure mentally while on the way to fetch the novice and gather supplies, if best use is to be made of the opportunity. Coordinators and instructors, of course, will need to plan for classes they are to teach.

Planning for instruction is done through use of the learning objectives, the written statements of expected changes in behavior as a result of learning. These changes can be in any or all the learning domains: cognitive, psychomotor, or affective.

As we have noted, objectives should be learner-centered, clear, and measurable. Each objective should state who is to perform the change in behavior, i.e., "The novice will . . ." or "The learner will . . ." rather than "To teach . . ." or "To review. . . ." Objectives should be clear and specific about what is expected of the learner.

When discussing planning for instruction with preceptors, it is a good idea to divide the procedure into two phases: macroplanning and microplanning. This helps to clarify responsibilities.

Macroplanning is planning on a large scale. This is the planning done by the program coordinator or head nurse that specifies an overall plan such as a residency program or a unit orientation. Objectives for the program will explain in detail what is to be accomplished during the program and cover activities on a daily, weekly, or monthly basis. Macroplans are often relatively specific and may also include what is to be done during a particular day or week.

Microplanning is done by the preceptor. This is planning on a smaller scale, for the hour, day, or week, to accomplish the goals and objectives outlined in the macroplan. Microplanning is just as important to a successful program as macroplanning. In fact, it may be more important, since it is through the microplans of the preceptor that larger objectives can be accomplished. Microplanning is the responsibility of the preceptor and facilitates learning on a day-to-day basis.

Teaching Principles

Several principles are important when discussing teaching and facilitating learning in addition to the ones discussed in the previous chapters. The following guidelines deal primarily with the sequencing of learning experiences.

Proceed from the simple to the complex. Don't try to cover the most complicated procedures first; build on the known to reach the unknown. Use terms and examples familiar to the novice.

Incorporate planned sequences of learning. Build on known skills or on a hierarchy to reach your goal. For example, preceptors might plan to show the novice how to do an admission in the morning and have the novice do the first admission for the afternoon, or coordinators may build on previously acquired physical assessment skills in a class on respiratory care.

Strive for immediate application. Try to cover material as it will be useful to the novice. For example, new graduates assigned to orthopedics obviously need to know the various types and purposes of traction setups. But instead of overwhelming the novice (and yourself) by trying to cover them all at once, incorporate the care of patients in various setups during the novice's stay on the unit. This brings the material into focus and allows immediate application of the information, which, in turn, enhances learning.

Be aware that content determines the kind of learning experience needed. It is impossible to effectively teach psychomotor skills unless practice time is included or problem solving if novices are never allowed to solve problems on their own. Think about the desired outcome and plan to incorporate experiences that will aid the novice in getting there. Exhibit 11-2 will assist you.

Don't forget the importance of positive reinforcement. We build on our successes, not our failures. Positive strokes help us to feel successful and to feel that we can go on to future learning. If the only comments we receive are negative ones, it is difficult to grow.

Once planning is complete, move to implement the plan. Again, remember the importance of small successes. Set small goals and encourage preceptors and novices to do the same. Success at reaching small goals encourages future striving and contributes to future success.

Teaching Techniques

Numerous teaching techniques and methods are available to carry out your plans. We will discuss some of the more common ones here. The Bibliography

Exhibit 11-2 Learning Activities and Objectives

		Desired Objectives	
	Cognitive	Affective	Psychomotor
Lecture	Yes	Can, if interesting	No
Discussion	Usually	Usually	No
Independent Study	Yes	Rarely	Can, if practice included
Demonstration	Yes	No	Yes
Practice	Can	Rarely	Yes
Role Play	No	Yes	Yes
Simulation	Can	Yes	Can
Games	Usually	No	No
Team Conferences	Yes	Can	No
Case Studies	Yes	Rarely	No
Process Recordings	Rarely	Yes	No
Care Plans	Yes	No	No

includes a variety of sources that cover these and others in more depth. Exhibit 11-3 outlines some of the advantages and disadvantages of various teaching methods.

Lecture

The lecture is probably the most common way of imparting information. Most of us are familiar with lectures from school and continuing education. While the lecture is a good way to impart large numbers of facts to groups of individuals, for the most part it is not the best method to incorporate into precepting. The lecture is a one-way communication, with one individual set up as the "expert" and the listeners as passive receptacles for information. There are better ways for preceptors to facilitate learning for novices.

Demonstration

The demonstration is frequently used in precepting. As activities, tasks, or procedures surface, the preceptor demonstrates for the novice the correct way of accomplishing the activities. When planning a demonstration, mentally run through each step of the procedure. If time permits, it is helpful to watch someone else doing the procedure and to jot down points you want stress. Gather the equipment you will need, and check to make sure that it works properly. Consider variations you wish to include, such as how one might do the procedure if the patient can't sit up or turn, or where scheduling forms are obtained when the

Exhibit 11-3 Learning Activities: Potential for Learner Involvement

	Maintains Interest	Motivating	Provides Immediate Feedback	Learner Proceeds at Own Rate
Lecture	Can, often fails	Can be	No	No
Discussion	Usually	Usually	Yes	Usually
Independent Study	Usually	Usually	Varies	Yes
Demonstration	Usually	Usually	Usually	Usually
Practice	Yes	Yes	Usually	Yes
Role Play	Yes	Usually	Yes	Usually
Simulation	Usually	Usually	Usually	Usually
Games	Usually	Yes	Yes	Usually
Team Conferences	Usually	Usually	Yes	Usually
Case Studies	Yes	Yes	Usually	Usually
Process recordings	Yes	Usually	Usually	Yes
Care Plans	Varies	Can be	No	Usually

staffing office is closed. Plan for practice time and a return demonstration to be sure that your points are understood and that the activity is performed correctly.

Team Conferences

Team conferences can be a useful format for imparting knowledge about particular disease entities, problems, or patients. Selected members of the nursing staff gather to discuss a particular patient and share information, strategies, and solutions. This works especially well when novices have patient situations they have difficulty dealing with and for which they need further information or solutions. Suggesting that the preceptor or novice arrange a team conference wherein solutions and assistance can be sought from other members of the staff gives novices experience in problem solving and in utilizing resource persons around them. It also pools information and gets the best thinking of those involved.

Case Studies

Case studies can be especially useful in settings where in-depth knowledge of a particular problem is desired, as they promote critical thinking and discrimination. This tutorial type of session allows the novice to explore, clarify confusions, and summarize thinking about a particular problem or patient, and it allows the instructor to probe and critically examine the novice's thinking patterns and problem-solving abilities. A comprehensive guideline for case study presentations is provided in Appendix H.

Simulation

Simulations provide realistic situations in which learners may practice requisite behaviors. Although simulations can be quite complicated to develop and run, they provide as close to a real a situation as possible without involving patients or staff. Most of us are familiar with simulations from the care we gave to dolls in the nursing fundamentals lab. Other common simulations involve cardiac arrest protocols or CPR skills.

Role Play

Role plays are a form of simulation in which hypothetical but realistic circumstances are developed and two or more individuals take the part of the persons involved. Role plays can illustrate points or provoke insights into another's viewpoint or position. Ground rules must be established and the end of the role play clearly defined so that the participants can step back into their normal roles and review the proceedings.

Process Recordings

Process recordings, verbatim notes of the novice's conversations with patients (or staff), allow reflection and analysis of person-to-person interactions. Process recordings can be especially useful when examination of approaches is necessary and alternative ways of interaction need to be considered. Although tape recordings provide a verbatim recall, often they are not practical and the novice must rely on memory. Process recordings or tape recordings are useful not only in analyzing interactions between individuals, but in assisting novices to give clearer, more concise reports or case presentations. Exhibit 11-4 provides one format for process recordings.

Independent Study

Independent study projects are helpful for novices. In conjunction with or at the instigation of the coordinator or preceptor, the novice decides that a particular topic is of interest. The novice researches the topic and presents findings. Objectives need to be spelled out clearly at the onset so that the coordinator, preceptor, and novice are all satisfied that the desired learning has occurred. A learning contract explicitly specifies objectives, responsibilities, and the evaluation format. Evaluation need not be written but may consist of a verbal report,

Exhibit 11-4 Process Recording Format

	Interaction	Feelings/Thoughts	Comments
Nurse:	"How are you feeling Mr. Jones?"	He looks like he's in pain.	
Patient:	"Not so hot."	Oh-Oh.	
Nurse:	"What's the matter?"	Must be his back.	
Patient:	"I hurt so much."	I thought so.	
Nurse:	"I'll get your pain med."		
Nurse:	"Here's your shot. Is the pain still in the same place in your back?"	I'm sure it is but just to be sure——.	
Patient:	"It's not my back, it's my chest. And I seem to be short of breath."	Good thing I asked—I need to take vital signs. Wonder if he's had chest pain before?	Next time I'll find out where the pain is *before* I go any further.

unit presentation, demonstration, or the like. A sample contract for an independent study project is shown in Exhibit 11-5.

Care Plans

Care plans are a useful teaching technique, as they force the novice to be specific about what is to be done and when. The why can then be explored by the preceptor and possible alternatives discussed. Care plans need not apply specifically to patients but may, for example, be a new manager's "care plan" for developing unit staff members.

Conducting incidental learning will probably comprise the bulk of the preceptor's time. Incidental learning consists of the small, individual items that come up during the day and about which the novice needs to be instructed. Where do you get the form needed? How do you contact the doctor? What will be asked about the patient? How often are staff evaluations to be done? When are schedules due at the nursing office? Most of the novices' questions will fall into this realm, and the experienced staff members will probably have little difficulty answering such questions.

Questioning

Good question-asking skills are essential for effective teaching. Questions stimulate learners to think and motivate further investigation and learning. Effective use of questioning involves five components: phrasing, delivery, wait-time, listening, and dealing with the response.

Phrasing of questions has much influence both on understanding and the type of responses you will receive. Open-ended questions, those that have no direct "yes" or "no" answer, will elicit more information and will allow better assessment of the learner. Consider the difference between "Do you know how to insert a Foley?" and "Tell me how you would insert a Foley in this patient," or "How many times have you inserted a Foley?"

Questions must be clear in their phrasing. How many times have you heard someone ask a question and then asked yourself "What does this person want to know?" Using language familiar to the novice, asking one question at a time, and being clear about what you are asking will help to elicit the information you are seeking.

Delivery of the question is important. If more than one learner is involved, address questions to the entire group and then ask for volunteers to answer or call on an individual. Encourage everyone's participation, not just those who volunteer. Also, encourage individual responses, instead of a chorus. This permits everyone to hear the answer given and minimizes confusion about the correct answer.

Exhibit 11-5 Contract for Independent Study

CONTRACT FOR INDEPENDENT STUDY

Topic Area: Hemodynamic monitoring: Swan-Ganz Catheters

Objectives:
1. Assemble and correctly set up equipment necessary for insertion of a Swan Ganz.

2. Describe nursing responsibility before, during, after insertion of a Swan Ganz.

3. Interpret normal from abnormal PAP, PCWP. State when you expect increased or decreased pressures. Identify appropriate nursing response to abnormal findings.

4. Correctly interpret and document pressures and waveforms.

Provisions: Will assist preceptor in care of at least 4 patients with S-G during contract period; evaluation date will be extended if insufficient number of patients with Swan Ganz.

Resources: Hemodynamic Monitoring Workshop on January 11th
Nursing Photobook on Monitoring
Policy and Procedure Book
Preceptor

Evaluation:

Date(s): On or before March 31st

Method: Demonstration; Question & Answer Session conducted by preceptor; monitored by Critical Care Specialist

Criteria:
1. Correctly assembles all equipment needed for insertion of Swan Ganz according to hospital policy.

2. Describes all nursing responsibility before, during and after insertion of Swan Ganz.

3. Demonstrates knowledge of normal from abnormal PAP, PCWP, when caring for patients and appropriate nursing actions. Able to identify expected deviations due to common disease conditions (left heart failure, COPD, pulmonary emboli, pulmonary edema, hypovolemia, tamponade).

4. Correctly documents findings according to hospital procedures.

Signatures_____

_____

Use waiting time effectively. This is difficult for new preceptors to learn, because there is a tendency to jump in immediately to prevent "that horrible silence." However, silence is necessary for learners to process questions and their potential responses. Try to consciously increase the time that you wait before expecting or asking for answers, and allow students time to think. If you find that the silence grates on your nerves, try counting to yourself "One-one-thousand, two-one-thousand" etc., allowing at least five seconds before you solicit responses.

Actively listen to the response you get. Maintain eye contact and pay attention to what is being said and how it is being communicated. Do not interrupt. Probe and explore the thinking behind the response if you need to. Be sure that the response is an adequate one before you move on to the next item.

What do you do when the response is not correct or is not the one you seek? Stress what is right about the response—"You're on the right track, take it a little further" or "You're right, in most instances that's true, but what about this particular case?" Ask for additional information. Avoid ridicule, sarcasm, or putting down the learner. You want to encourage active participation, not inhibit it.

TEACHING PITFALLS

Novice behaviors sometimes cause difficulties for instructors or preceptors. You should be aware of the more common ones and possible ways to handle them.

Sidetracking

Sidetracking can be a major difficulty for new instructors. The learner desires to escape an anxiety-provoking situation, such as trying a new procedure for the first time, and sidesteps the issue by indirect means—perhaps becoming "too busy" to try the new procedure or asking a multitude of tangentially related questions. The preceptor or instructor must be aware that this is happening and redirect the topic to the original issue. If the behavior persists, the reasons behind the behavior must be explored and aired.

Anxiety

Being led into the novice's anxiety system can also be difficult for new preceptors or instructors to avoid. Anxiety is catching, and it is possible to pick it up from our learners. This becomes a vicious circle for as our own anxiety increases so does that of our students. Soon we are trapped in an escalating spiral. Particularly as new preceptors or instructors we are anxious about our own performance. The student's anxiety leads us to question whether we are being too hard or expecting too much. Sort out your own anxieties from those of the learner, and don't be caught by their anxieties.

Try not to spend exorbitant amounts of time trying to untangle a learner's thinking. Certainly, we need to clear up misunderstandings, but if it becomes obvious that untangling the web will be a lengthy undertaking, other options and resources need to be sought to assist the learner.

Be careful of locking into one solution of a problem. Often we wear blinders and become oblivious to the multiplicity of options available. Any problem has numerous solutions, and chances are that several of them are equally good. We choose the one we prefer based on past experience and our value system. Often our learners will choose other alternatives. Before automatically correcting them, stop and think for a moment. Is their solution really below par, or is our own choice of a solution being imposed on them? Often, upon examination, the latter is the case.

Another frequent delusion for new instructors or preceptors is the feeling that we must have all the answers. As we have noted, to be effective, you need not have all the answers. Frequently, you are more effective if you don't since this allows the novices to see that they need not know everything. As the old adage goes, "It's not whether you know it or not, but whether you know where to get it that matters." When we admit that we don't have all the answers, it frees our novices to admit to similar gaps.

Do not allow yourself to be pushed into making decisions for the novice or student. Show respect for the novice's ability to make a good decision, and serve as a sounding board instead of making the decision for the novice. If you are uncomfortable with the conclusion, ask leading questions in an effort to redirect thinking. "Have you thought about . . ." or "What about . . ." can help learners to reassess their conclusions while developing their confidence in their ability to make decisions.

One of the most difficult things for preceptors to do is to let go of their novices, to allow them the freedom to do things on their own, make decisions on their own, and take responsibility for those activities and decisions. There is no easy answer to this. Each person must find his or her own way of letting go. Some preceptors put distance between their novices and themselves. Some talk themselves into letting go.

Stage fright is a common experience for preceptors and new instructors alike. The idea of teaching others, of being the expert, is overwhelming. As many preceptors put it, "I've still got so much to learn myself. How can I possibly have something to teach others? I get sick to my stomach just thinking about it."

Nervous stomachs, feeling faint, palpitations, or clumsiness hit when we least expect it or when it seems most humiliating. Ranging from mere jitters to overwhelming terror, stage fright strikes us all.

As scary as stage fright is, we need to recognize that we are not alone in our feelings. Most of us have at least some degree of stage fright when we must address others. There are ways to make it less terrorizing.

First, admit that you're scared. Try to pinpoint exactly what it is about the experience that frightens you. Perhaps it is a fear of forgetting what you are to say, or of tripping on your way to the podium. Or a fear of sounding dumb. Whatever it is, once identified it becomes easier to deal with.

Separate your performance as a speaker or teacher from yourself as a person. Regardless of whether the performance is a roaring success or a resounding disaster, you are a worthwhile, multifaceted individual. Your intrinsic worth will not be changed by the results of your performance. Prepare thoroughly. Research your material if you can. Rehearse mentally what you will say and how you will say it. Think of logical questions and figure out how you would answer them. Picture your worst fears and decide what you would do if they happened. What will you say and do if you DO trip on your way to the stage? How would you respond to hecklers? How will you help yourself remember what to say? Most of our fears never come true, but you will feel much more prepared if you have considered the possibilities before and have figured out how you will respond.

Anticipate the positive. Concentrate on the good things: questions mean that the individuals who heard you were really interested in what you had to say; hecklers allow you an opportunity to restate your position if it wasn't clear. Think how you will feel when people really hear what you are saying.

Be good to yourself. Get plenty of rest, exercise, and eat well. Cut down on caffeine. Find a reward for yourself when you have finished your task—a walk in the woods, a hot fudge sundae, whatever. Treat yourself well and you will be better prepared for whatever happens.

EVALUATING TEACHING AND LEARNING

Once your plan for teaching is completed and has been implemented, you are ready to evaluate whether it was successful. Clear, concise objectives are a great help here, as they outline exactly what the learner must accomplish. Review each objective jointly with the learner and decide whether or not the objective has been met. Often this will be easy. A successful return demonstration, a verbal review of material—whatever method is appropriate for the objective will suffice. The review need not be all at one time; if you watched the novice successfully perform a technique previously, obviously it does not have to be repeated unless you are uncomfortable about the novice's ability to recall information or discriminate between instances. Refer to Chapters 8 and 14 for more extensive discussion of evaluation.

SUMMARY

This chapter has considered teaching—what makes successful teachers, teaching methods, and common problems. Our next chapter will move on to an essential of effective teaching—clear communication.

REFERENCES

Conley, V. (1973). *Curriculum and instruction in nursing.* Boston: Little, Brown.

Knowles, M.S. (1970). *The modern practice of adult education.* New York: Association Press.

Chapter 12

Communication

Effective communication is essential in all realms of life. It is especially important to both nursing preceptors and coordinators, where the conveyance of information from one individual to another is crucial. This chapter concentrates on productive communication.

We normally think of communication as a verbal medium. Yet communication really embraces all methods of information transmittal, including gestures, signs, writing, body language, and cues.

The process of communication involves one individual sending a message to another with the intention of stimulating a response. The three crucial elements are (1) a sender, (2) a receiver, and (3) a message, which may be either verbal or nonverbal. Full, effective interchange requires that the receiver fully understand the message intended by the sender.

Sender, receiver, message. The process would seem to be a very simple one. Why is it, then, that effective communication is so rare and so difficult to achieve?

THE SENDER-RECEIVER INTERCHANGE

A number of factors influence the sender-receiver interchange. These affect the clarity of the message and determine the receiver's interpretation of the message.

The Verbal Element

A major determinant for verbal messages are the words used. When the message is verbal, the words used are crucial. Each of us makes a personal set of pictures from the words others use. These pictures vary, depending on our background and experiences. For example, what picture do you get from the word "house"? To some, it conjures up a Victorian, Georgian, or contemporary structure. To others, Dutch Colonial, medieval Tudor, or modern A-frame images appear. Some will picture the inside rather than the outside of the house, or the people living there.

Words are used to hide or express emotions and to express social conventions. Often we don't really want meaningful answers to conventional social politenesses. When asked "How are you?" most of us will respond out of habit or convention "Fine," even though we may not be feeling well.

Words change their meaning with context, with geographical location, over time, and in response to social events and developments. Meaning changes in different parts of the country. To New Yorkers and Seattleites, a milkshake contains ice cream. To Bostonians, a milkshake is flavored milk; to get ice cream one asks for a frappe. Abbreviations likewise change, even among our own subculture of medicine. Someone from the northeast might be unfamiliar with I.S. (incentive spirometer). A colleague from the northwest can be unfamiliar with AAA (abdominal aortic aneurysm).

Words and meanings evolve over time to meet societal needs. Different cultures and subcultures have their own words, frequently unfamiliar to those outside. Bankers, doctors, and financiers are frequently accused of not speaking English. The same might be said for musicians, nurses, and artists. Multiple minicultures exist as well. Cardiovascular nurses, for example, use terms and abbreviations unfamiliar to renal or orthopedic nurses, and vice versa. Novices learn, in time, to speak the language of their subculture. Instructors of novices must be careful to translate unfamiliar words and phrases.

The Nonverbal Element

Even when we are actively using words to express our messages, a substantial part of our communication takes place on a nonverbal level.

Personal Space

Personal space is a result of defining one's territory. Each of us defines several personal bubbles of space for ourselves. These concentric rings determine comfortable distances for interactions. Hall (1969) defines four distances: the intimate, from 0 to approximately one and a half feet; the personal, from one and a half feet to four feet; the social, from four to twelve feet; and the public, from twelve feet on. We give permission for those we are intimate with, such as family members, to enter our personal space but become uncomfortable when others do so without our permission. Those who enter our space without our permission convey a message of threat to us, and we back away or terminate the conversation.

Body Language

Body posture, movements, and gestures reflect an unspoken message and reveal underlying feelings and attitudes. Unconscious finger tapping reveals nervousness or impatience with what's being said; crossed arms are a sign that the listener is closed to the conversation. Facial expressions convey a whole range of emotions through slight changes in muscle position. Astute observers can pick up on these signals and pursue more meaningful communication as a result of their interpretation of the messages being sent.

Visual Interaction

Overall appearance often encapsulates an underlying message: "I'm clean, neat, and well groomed; I care about myself and others." We draw immediate inferences about the individual who appears before us with hair uncombed, unshaven, and in slovenly dress and interpret their messages with that image in mind.

Eye contact and facial expressions are important parts of visual interaction. Embarrassment, guilt, and aggression are frequently read in others through the type and degree of eye contact. The person who meets another's eyes openly and directly conveys a different message than the person who cannot meet another's look directly and shifts his or her gaze away. An entire message can be encapsulated in a facial expression. The happy, animated face of good news varies considerably from the down-turned, solemn face of bad. Often you need not even hear the verbal message to make the correct interpretation.

Vocalization

Vocalization includes the ability to speak as well as the vocal tone, stress, and patterns. An inability to adequately vocalize carries multiple difficulties. The laryngectomy patient who has not yet adequately relearned speech has a difficult and frustrating time being understood. Accents may affect understanding in a similar manner. Everyone has, at one time or another, had difficulty understanding those from other parts of the country or from other nations. The words are the same but the speed, patterns, stress, and tone change, garbling the message received.

Tones carry an underlying message of their own. They convey authority or impotence, sadness or exhilaration, or the degree of control of feelings. Our culture teaches us to change the tone with our mood or certain situations. Questions end with a raised tone. This cues the listener, nonverbally, that a response is needed. Questions asked without that change in tone are often ignored. Messages in a monotone carry one underlying connotation; those in a high, squeaky pitch another. There are times when a room of people suddenly becomes hushed when a deeply toned voice asks for quiet although a shrill pitch was unable to achieve silence only a moment before. The message remained the same, only the tone changed. Occasionally, words give one message, the tone another. This incongruence confuses the receiver and the intended message may be lost. The expert communicator listens to both messages and explores for the true one.

Changes in the stress of words are also important. Consider the differences between "*Call* me in the morning," "Call *me* in the morning," and "Call me in the *morning*." The words remain the same; the message changes depending on the words stressed.

Setting

The setting may either enhance or inhibit the clarity of the message. Appropriateness of setting is important. The environment suitable for a social chat would be inappropriate for an evaluation and vice versa. In addition, noise, lighting, temperature, and ventilation can be important influences. The setting must be appropriate and without distractions if the listener is to really hear, understand, and act upon the message.

Expectations

Sender and receiver expectations affect message clarity. The subtle message will not be clear to the listener who expects to be told bluntly. It simply won't be heard. Likewise, the person tuned in to the subtle or covert message will feel overwhelmed by the bluntness needed by the first listener.

Expectations color all of our communications. We hear what we expect to hear—not what is actually said. Our presumptions regarding the speaker, the topic, and the position to be taken by the speaker distort the intent of the speaker's message. In some cases, we reprogram the sender's message to make it more in line with what we expected, what we want, or what is more congruent with our own beliefs, values, or opinions.

Congruence

Congruence is essential for a clear understanding of any message. Congruence is disturbed when the verbal and nonverbal elements of communication don't match, when the words say one thing and the nonverbal elements (tone of voice and appearance, for example) say something else. Consider what happens when the answer to your question is "yes," accompanied by turning of the head from side-to-side. In addition, what one says is not necessarily what one implies. For example, "I'm not disagreeing with you" often implies you're doing exactly that. Incongruence between elements of the communication disturbs the meaning of the message and confuses the receiver.

Receiver Involvement

Receiver involvement in the interaction is essential to be sure that the intended message was received. This is particularly crucial in one-to-one or small group interactions. Feedback ensures that understanding has occurred. It may be verbal or nonverbal; often a facial expression is far more evocative of the recipient's reaction than verbal feedback could possibly be. But verbal feedback permits full exchange and questions—essential if the message is complex.

COMMUNICATION TOOLS

Murray and Zentner (1975) identify five tools for communication: language, observation and perception, silence, and listening. Effective application of these tools is essential to productive communication.

Language

Obviously, language is basic to communication. Without the ability to translate pictures into symbols and have those symbols understood by others, the ability to transfer thoughts from one person to another is severely hampered. Those who cannot speak the same language often experience a frustration equal to those who cannot speak at all.

Observation and Perception

Observation and perception are important because so much of our translation of messages relies on nonverbal elements. Without the ability to observe the speaker's appearance and translate observed body language, we are hindered in our attempt to fully interpret the message, its motivation, and its intent.

Silence

Silence is an exceedingly powerful tool in communication. A productive silence occurs when the listener is thinking through a problem or reflecting upon what was said. Nonproductive silences occur when the listener is bored with or disinterested in the topic of conversation. Silences may also occur when the listener is embarrassed, feels apprehensive or fearful, or is unsure of the listeners' acceptance of his or her message.

Listening

Listening is an important tool in communication. Active listening is essential for full and effective message sending and receiving. Active listening requires availability, attentiveness, and acceptance (Rowland & Rowland, 1980).

Availability is essential if you are to be a good listener. This means that you are at the disposal of the speaker when he or she needs to talk, that you are willing to hear what the speaker has to say in meetings, impromptu discussion, and formal presentations.

Attentiveness means that you give speakers your full attention, that you do not allow your mind to wander to other matters while someone is speaking. This requires receptivity both verbally, demonstrated through the use of encouragers such as "go on," and nonverbally, using your tone, body language, and visual cues to express your involvement and interest in what is being said.

Finally, to be a good listener you must demonstrate acceptance of what is being said. Try to understand where speakers are coming from and not prejudge what they are going to say. Allow them to freely express their thoughts and opinions; don't correct, argue, or harass them. Offer your perspective as an alternative view only after the sender has finished speaking. A nonjudgmental and accepting approach will help speakers to more clearly express their ideas and will leave them more open to hearing your alternative views and opinions. Exhibit 12-1 contains a self-evaluation of listening habits.

PROBLEMS IN COMMUNICATION

Now we come directly to some of the common problems encountered in communicating with others. Understanding these communication blocks can help you to present your own messages in the clearest, most nonthreatening way possible. We shall discuss a number of blocks but begin with an examination of defensiveness, since raising the other person's defenses is one of the most common problems encountered in our attempts to communicate.

Defensiveness

Defensive people spend a majority of their energies defending themselves: analyzing how they appear to others, how they may find favor, and how they can control, dominate, impress, and avoid or minimize a perceived or anticipated attack. Defensive behavior becomes a vicious circle. The attempts to protect oneself lead to defensive listening. This generates defensive verbal and nonverbal cues, which in turn raise the defense level of the sender. Defensive communication prevents the listener from focusing on the message. It distorts reception, and listeners are less able to accurately perceive the emotions, motives, and values of the sender.

Gibb (1961) identified six categories of defensive-supportive communication. These are evaluation-description, control-problem orientation, strategy-spontaneity, neutrality-empathy, superiority-equality, and certainty-provisionalism.

Exhibit 12-1 Evaluation of Listening Habits

1. I listen by conscientiously focusing my thoughts on the person who is speaking to me and what they are saying, and commit myself to really listen.
2. I begin asking questions about what I heard before letting the other person know what I heard or understood.
3. I listen to the person by watching eyes, face, body posture, movement, and listening to other voice cues.
4. I analyze and try to interpret for myself what the other person is saying rather than asking for clarification of what I thought I heard or understood him/her to say.
5. I listen for what *is not* being said as well as for what *is* being said.
6. I think about other things, daydream, plan my evening, etc. while "listening" to the other person.
7. I show in a physical way that I am listening and interested, and I try to help the other person feel comfortable in sharing with me.
8. I often act like I am listening even when I am not, especially when I am busy or feel I already know what the person is going to say.
9. I am aware of the listening or non-listening cues I am giving to the other person such as facial, body, and vocal cues.
10. I listen for particular words or phrases or detail more than I listen for the overall ideas of the person to whom I am listening.
11. I use mirror responses to feed back to the person specific words or phrases he/she has used that I need clarified.
12. I interrupt with my own personal "I've been there" story by making comments such as "I know just what you mean" or "That's happened to me, too," and then going on to tell my story before letting the other person finish, or before letting them know that I heard and understood what they were saying, feeling, etc.
13. I paraphrase or summarize what I heard the other person saying before giving my own personal feeling or point of view.
14. I think of what I am going to say next before the person has finished speaking.
15. I consistently ask for feedback to verify my perception of the other person's message.
16. I am easily distracted by noises and/or the speaker's manner of delivery.

Now read your list.

Place a check in front of each habit you have (even if you only use that habit sometimes).

Next, reread the habits you placed checks in front of and place a + in front of all the habits that you perform while listening almost all of the time (75–100).

Now, in the spaces provided below, place an X by each number you have indicated by a plus.

MOST INEFFECTIVE LISTENING HABITS

2. ___
4. ___
6. ___
8. ___
10. ___
12. ___
14. ___
16. ___

MOST EFFECTIVE LISTENING HABITS

1. ___
3. ___
5. ___
7. ___
9. ___
11. ___
13. ___
15. ___

Exhibit 12-1 continued

Now that you have an inventory of your most effective and ineffective listening habits, you may want to establish priorities of those habits you wish to eliminate and those you wish to develop or strengthen.

THREE LISTENING HABITS I WISH TO ELIMINATE ARE:

1. _____

2. _____

3. _____

THREE LISTENING HABITS I WISH TO STRENGTHEN OR DEVELOP:

1. _____

2. _____

3. _____

Source: Cheryl Kilbourn. Reprinted by permission.

The first term describes the defensive behavior, the second the supportive behavior.

Speech that is interpreted as evaluative puts one on the defensive. It implies that a value judgment is being made and puts the receiver on guard. A less defense-provoking technique to use is an information-seeking approach. This minimizes the reflexive personal protectiveness and promotes more open communication.

A controlling approach indicates a desire and an attempt to change another. It implies inadequacies in the receiver, thereby raising one's defenses. An approach that emphasizes mutual collaboration to solve problems will be received more favorably than one that attempts to impose control. This permits each individual to bring his or her own values and creativity to the problem and promotes a true exchange of ideas.

If the sender is perceived as using certain strategies to achieve his or her own ends, it promotes defensiveness and resentfulness on the part of the receiver. We feel resistance to those who try to manipulate us, particularly if the assumption on their part seems to be that we are too naive to see the underlying motivation. If the sender is seen as spontaneous and straightforward, with open motivations, communications will be received more favorably.

Empathy is important in communication if the receiver is not to become defensive. Empathy implies a concern for the individual who is sending the message and conveys warmth and respect. The totally neutral person is interpreted as uncaring and is not seen as supportive.

Conveying superiority engenders defensiveness. The individual who implies that he or she is above others in any way (intelligence, wealth, physical appearance, power, etc.) tells the listener that the listener is inadequate and that therefore the sender is unwilling to participate in any activity (such as mutual problem solving) on an equal footing. The person who implies equality from the beginning will find his or her messages more favorably received.

Certainty also engenders defensiveness. Those who already know the answers need no help or information from others. Often combined with controlling communication, certainty makes effective transmittal of ideas difficult at best. When one is open minded and willing to explore new ideas, defensiveness is reduced.

The Environment

As mentioned previously, the environment can be a major deterrent to effective communication. Anyone who has tried to converse in a noisy hallway, restaurant, or office knows how little of the message can be heard. Smells, inadequate lighting, and uncomfortable temperatures may also interfere with senders sending adequate messages and receivers correctly interpreting them.

Attitude

The sender's attitude can inhibit communication. Individuals who come across as evaluative, superior, or dogmatic, for example, effectively shut off communication from others.

Ambivalence

Ambivalence is a common block. The individual who vacillates between positive and negative feelings at the same time may express both emotions. Unless the receiver is aware of the ambivalence or can help the sender explore it, the message conveyed may be far from the correct one, although it may be reflective of true feelings at the moment it is said. Incongruence between reality and values and expectations often engenders ambivalence and is relatively common in novices.

Reassurance

Reassurance can be a block to communication since it effectively prohibits further communication. Common reassurances such as "Everything will be all right" convey the opinion from the sender that the emotions and anxieties of the receiver are unimportant and close off further exchange.

Rejection of Ideas

Rejection of ideas also blocks communication. The common lists of ten (or one hundred) reasons "Why It Can't Be Done" reflect how frequently ideas are refused without fair hearing. This of course inhibits further communications from both that individual and others. "There's no point in suggesting anything; it'll just get shot down." No one likes rejection and few will choose to experience it needlessly.

Activity

A common block to communication for nurses is the myth that a good nurse is a busy nurse. We feel guilty ourselves and denigrate our colleagues for taking time to sit and listen. We must always be doing something. Yet to be effective listeners we must take the time to really hear what is being said. To be effective preceptors, we must take the time to sit down and explore what is happening with our novice. Unfortunately, this badly needed communication occurs rarely if at all, taking a back seat to the never-ending flow of tasks. Too often, we seem convinced that unless we are actively doing tasks we are not doing our job. In reality, often the opposite is true.

Talk

An inability to tolerate silence is a block to communication. Silence allows reflection and a pulling together of thoughts. If constantly interrupted, this consolidation of thinking cannot take place and important synthesis may be lost. The ability to wait and allow the listener time for reflection is essential for an effective interchange.

Sermonettes block communication. This preaching, laced with shoulds and oughts, inhibits further exchange as individuals become tired of being told what they should or should not do, think, or feel. Sermonettes are frequently a defensive response to a challenge to one's value or belief system and they in turn engender a defensive response.

"War stories" are another block to communication. While potentially useful for illustrating a particular point, too often such stories of past exploits and experiences serve only to subtly illustrate the sender's superiority.

IMPROVING COMMUNICATION

How can you improve communication with others or assist others to improve their communication? Several strategies are available. We shall start with a discussion of question asking, as this is one of the most common methods of facilitating communication between two parties.

Questions

Ask direct questions. Such questions provide feedback to the sender about the clarity of the message and allow an opportunity for clarification and elaboration.

If you as a receiver are unsure about the message or desire more information, ask for it. Often the receiver hears only part of an intended message. Be certain all of the message has been received and that it has been clearly understood. As a sender, ask questions to be sure that receivers hear the intended message and that their interpretations are correct.

Use open-ended questions, those that cannot be answered with a clear-cut "yes" or "no," to seek clarification. These promote further exchange and convey openness and an interest in both what is said and the sender.

Utilize small talk when needed. While social chatter is frequently inhibiting to an open exchange, it serves as an icebreaker or breather period in some cases. A minute or two of chitchat can help to reduce tension and set the tone. You can then proceed to deeper levels of exchange. Care must be taken not to overuse this technique or to use it in times of high emotion when it will be perceived as avoidance.

Confront others when necessary, but take care to choose your times carefully, as confrontation may either inhibit or enhance communication. Effective confrontation, a laying of cards out on the table, must be followed by mutual problem solving. One approach is to confront, then to ask what can be done about it. "Jane, this is the third time this week that you've forgotten Mr. Smith's 11 a.m. medication. What can we do to help you remember?" Approached in this manner, confrontation becomes the basis for cooperation rather than conflict.

Seek clarification so that both parties clearly understand the messages. Such statements as "I'm not sure I quite understand what you mean" or "Do you mean . . ." help to clarify messages for both sender and receiver. Occasionally, summarize what has been said or the other's main points in your own words and give him or her a chance to correct any misunderstandings.

Encouraging comparisons between situations can be especially helpful. Statements and questions such as "How is this like . . ." help the other person reflect upon past experiences and relate knowledge or skills gained to the current situation. This promotes communication as it allows the receiver to seek his or her own solution while providing a framework within which to do so.

Feedback

Providing feedback is crucial if communication between two individuals is to be clear. Assumptions and inferences frequently distort our understanding. Only by giving and receiving frequent and effective feedback can you be sure that the messages are clear and that understanding occurs. Use reflective responses to encourage elaboration and promote self-exploration and thought. "It sounds as if you're really angry at your school. . . ." This approach helps the individual explore thoughts and feelings and provides an accepting atmosphere in which to express oneself.

Acknowledging feelings and thoughts validates your involvement in the exchange. "Yes" or "I hear what you're saying" communicates both that you've understood what was said and your interest in continuing the communication. This enhances further communication.

Express doubt where appropriate. Full and effective communication does not imply agreement with everything that is said. Be careful in your wording not to censure, ridicule, or argue, which promotes defensiveness and reduces communication effectiveness. Instead try to provoke alternative ways of thinking about the topic. Statements such as "Is that really your conclusion?" and "Do you really think that is what is happening in this case?" promote self-exploration. The message conveyed is that not all persons see the situation in the same way, nor do all draw the same conclusions.

Verbalize the implied. Follow up on what is hinted at. Too often we assume we understand the reference only to later discover otherwise. This garbles the message and confuses our interpretation. In addition, such subtle references are often cues to what is really thought or felt. Unless such inferences are explored, the feelings behind them cannot be fully resolved. Mutterings under the breath such as "They never told me it would be like this" are important cues to underlying emotions. Once out in the open, they can be confronted, defused, and dealt with appropriately.

Encouragers are also important. They convey concern and a genuine interest in what is being said. "Go on" or "Tell me more" reinforces your involvement in the topic and with the speaker and supports further communication.

In all of these techniques, focus on specifics. Global phrases such as "all," "none," or "no one" confuse rather than clarify. "You always do that" is not the best approach. Concentrate on specific situations, persons, or examples to define particulars and promote precise interpretations.

ASSERTIVE AND AGGRESSIVE BEHAVIOR

Much has been said and written over the past five years about assertive and aggressive behaviors. Since interpretations of what is assertive rather than aggressive rest on communication styles, we shall take a few moments to examine these styles here.

There are basically four styles of communication: assertive, nonassertive, aggressive, and passive-aggressive. Assertive and aggressive communication have often been defined as opposites, assertive implying "good," aggressive implying hostile or "bad" communication.

Bakker and Bakker-Rabdau (1973), in *No Trespassing! Explorations in Human Territoriality*, dispel these labels of good and bad. By defining assertiveness and aggressiveness in a territorial model, they help to clarify both. A territory, they say, is "any object of territorial behavior. It may be a stretch of land, an idea, a function or anything else that holds a person's fancy to such a degree that he seeks to own it" (p. 271). Territorial behavior is the "set of observable behaviors which an individual consistently exhibits relative to any concrete or abstract area. Such behaviors include efforts to gain control over an area, actions to mark the area in order to proclaim ownership, and defense of the area against intruders" (p. 271).

The purpose of assertiveness is to retain or regain control over a disputed area and effectively rebuff the aggressor. Specific forms of assertiveness may include verbal ("Get off my foot") or nonverbal responses (removing your foot from underneath and nudging the other person's back).

Aggression seeks to expand those territories already owned. It implies active pursuit and exploration, rather than hostility. In other words, any behavior that leads to enlargement, no matter how temporary, of territories can be labeled aggressive. In the example given above, nudging the other person's foot back farther than its original placement could be considered aggressive.

Hostility, on the other hand, is "behavior which seeks to destroy or injure an individual or his territory" (Bakker & Bakker-Rabdau, 1973, p. 269). Hostility need not be recognized as such by the perpetrator:

> If the distinction is to be made on what people say about their intention, one is in real trouble, for human beings are masters of deceiving themselves as well as others . . . the judgment as to whether any behavior seeks to destroy, on the one hand, or acquire new territory, on the other, must be made on the basis of observed behavior and its consequences. (Bakker & Bakker-Rabdau, 1973, p. 63)

An inability to be assertive almost always leads to hostility. It is this retaliatory hostile behavior, rather than aggressive behavior, that we should seek to avoid.

Assertive or aggressive communication tries to openly and honestly convey true feelings and opinions. It supports the individual and his or her rights without hindering the rights of others. For example, you've assigned your novice Mr. X to take care of today. The novice reminds you that she took care of Mr. X last week and feels quite comfortable now in doing so but would like to take Mrs. Z as she has several dressings and tubes that the novice is still uncomfortable with. The novice openly and honestly seeks to expand territorial areas of expertise but does so without dominating others and remains open to your advice and rationale.

In contrast is the nonassertive communicator. This individual is afraid to assert his or her own needs and wants and passively submits to others. He or she takes on Mr. X's care, but silently resents not getting the learning experience truly needed and desired

Hostile communication again takes two forms: the overt and the covert. Hostile communicators seek to destroy. They are pushy and combative in their approach, intending to meet their own needs even at the expense of others. The hostile novice lets you know, in an aggressive and belligerent way, that she'll take Mrs. Z regardless of your wishes, advice, or rationale in the matter. She has nothing to learn from Mr. X. You're left fuming and in doubt about who is in control.

Covert hostility produces passive aggressiveness. Individuals who operate in this mode resemble nonassertive communicators in that they are unable or unwilling to make their needs and wants known but they rebel indirectly. The covertly hostile novice takes on the care of Mr. X but "forgets" important medications or treatments or conveys her unwillingness to do so in her attitude toward the patient and other staff.

Coordinators must help preceptors and novices to understand these concepts and to apply them. Assertiveness is appropriate in situations where one desires to maintain territory; aggression in those where one desires to gain territory. The use of assertive behavior when one attempts to add territory inhibits rather than enhances the chances for success. An inability to be assertive leaves individuals unable to respond appropriately, and they must resort to defensiveness or hostility.

Guidelines

Several rules of thumb can help troubled communicators turn their efforts in a more assertive direction. First, personalize your requests. Use "I" rather than "you." The use of "I" promotes understanding and minimizes the possibilities of alienating others. Listen to the difference between "I need that patient ready for X-ray at 11 a.m." and "You have that patient ready for X-ray at 11 a.m." The "I" makes quite a difference.

Second, be brief and specific. Outline what you need, the time limit, and consequences, if they apply, in your mind before you speak. "If we are to have Mr. Jones ready for surgery at 10 a.m., I need you to give his medications now." Be clear about what you need, and let others know.

Be persistent. It may take repeated statements and rephrasings of the same idea before it is clear you were really heard. Don't give up in your attempts. In our example of the assertive novice, she may have needed to repeat her preference for Mrs. Z over Mr. X, reiterating her feeling that working with Mrs. Z would be a better learning experience, several times before she was really heard.

If you are being aggressive rather than assertive, be prepared to give in gracefully. You haven't lost anything; you didn't have it to begin with. If territories are to be gained, the risk of being rebuffed by an assertive individual must be taken. Nothing ventured, nothing gained.

Disclose your feelings. This helps others to understand where you are coming from. Statements such as "I feel we are making a mistake here" or "I'm really angry about this incident" express and underscore your feelings and opinions but do not inhibit others from expressing theirs. Listen carefully for the truth and agree with it. Often the truth becomes buried in a morass of detail. Don't be afraid to outline and highlight it.

Recognize and admit when you're wrong. We all make mistakes. You'll be better respected for your ability to admit your fallibility than you will be if you are never wrong. Assertiveness doesn't mean that you can't change your mind or make a mistake. It just means that you aren't willing to be walked on.

Get feedback from others. If a particularly difficult exchange is witnessed by someone else, discuss the incident with that person. Get his or her opinion of the interaction and explore other strategies or approaches you might have used to enhance the communication.

Finally, set your limits and stick to them. Decide what you need, or clarify from others what they need. An example: Your head nurse, Mrs. Jones, stops you in the hall and says that Mrs. A is on her way to the floor and you should drop everything and admit her. You are about to start Mr. T's lengthy dressing procedure, which must be done on time. Your response to Mrs. Jones: "I'd be glad to, but I'm about to start Mr. T's dressing. Do you want me to delay the dressing for an hour?" This sets the limits of what you can reasonably accomplish and defines who is responsible for priority setting.

SUMMARY

Effective communication is essential for program staff, preceptors, and novices. This chapter has covered the basics of communication. Like any other skill, effective communication takes constant practice. The next chapter will move into one form of communication in action—supervising others.

REFERENCES

Bakker, C.B., & Bakker-Rabdau, M.K. (1973). *No Trespassing! Explorations in human territoriality.* San Francisco: Chandler and Sharp.

Gibb, J.R. (1961). Defensive communication. *Journal of Communication, 11*(3), 141–148.

Hall, E.T. (1969). *The hidden dimension.* Garden City, NY: Anchor Books/Doubleday.

Murray, R., & Zentner, J. (1975). *Nursing concepts for health promotion.* Englewood Cliffs, NJ: Prentice-Hall.

Rowland H.S., & Rowland, B.L. (1980). *Nursing administration handbook.* Rockville, MD: Aspen Systems.

Chapter 13

Supervision

This chapter begins our discussion of supervision in precepting. Why address supervision in a book on precepting?

According to the Washington State Practical Nurse Practice Act, supervision is the "critical evaluation of acts, performed with authority to take corrective action, but shall not be construed so as to require direct and bodily presence." (RCW 1818.78.010) Preceptors supervise their novices since they both critically evaluate acts and have the authority to take corrective action. Similarly, coordinators supervise both novices and preceptors.

In their role as supervisors, coordinators and preceptors should concentrate on the positive aspects of performance rather than the negative. Smoyak (1978) discusses the value of coaching as an approach instead of the more common one of telling people what they do wrong. Coaching should be the basis of precepting if individuals are to be helped to develop in the desired directions.

Coaching is the use of positive feedback to enhance and reinforce behavior that we desire continued. The ability to recognize small aspects of behavior we desire and encourage them while ignoring negative behaviors works to enhance self-esteem and create a positive environment for growth. It is this approach that should be encouraged.

Inherent in this approach is the assumption that we start with what people can do, not with what the job requires. Any nursing position is a mixture of complex interpersonal and technical skills. We enter new positions with both strengths and limitations. It is important to build on and reinforce the strengths, concentrating on how they enhance performance in the new role, rather than focusing on what the new individual cannot do. This does not mean being blind to weaknesses, but rather refraining from focusing on them unless they are hindering effective performance.

LEADERSHIP

Supervision involves leadership. In actuality, we are all leaders just as we are all followers. We move from leader to follower roles depending on the situation, its context, and our mood. Often we are leaders in one setting, followers in another. For example, at work we may be a leader, at home more of a follower; or we may be leaders in orthopedic care, followers in cardiovascular. None of us is a leader in all settings and situations.

When we think of leadership, we often think of the traditional, rather simplistic categories of autocratic, democratic, and laissez-faire leadership styles. Autocratic styles are those in which the leader makes all the decisions and the followers merely obey orders; democratic leadership involves more consultative and participatory styles; and laissez-faire, the "let them alone" style of some managers, abdicates a formal leadership role (Hersey & Blanchard, 1982, p. 87). The connotation is that democratic leadership is inherently good and autocratic and laissez-faire leadership are inferior.

In reality, this is not true. The style of leadership called for depends on the situation. Crises or emergencies call for autocratic management; this is not the time to gather views and consult. Imagine the chaos if each time a cardiac arrest was announced the head nurse gathered the staff and discussed possible options to reach consensus about what should be done. On the other hand, there are times when participative styles of leadership are needed. When acceptance of a decision by followers is critical to effective implementation, when conflict is likely, or when followers share in the responsibility for making the decision happen, it is best to include them in the decision-making process (Vroom & Yetten, 1973). Consistency in leadership style is behaving in the same way in similar situations for all parties concerned, not the blanket application of one leadership style to the exclusion of others. Vroom and Yetten's model for decision making can be of assistance in deciding which approach is best for a particular situation.

MOTIVATION

Leading consists of motivating others as well as making decisions. What is motivation? Webster (1967) defines it as "something (a need or desire) that causes a person to act." This definition is fine as far as it goes. But what need or desire? Researchers have been trying to answer that question for a long time. Generally, theories of motivation fall into four categories (Murray, 1964).

Cognitive Theories

Cognitive theories presume that persons act because they think they should do so or refuse to act because they believe they should not. Until Freud, it was commonly accepted that as rational beings humans controlled their own motivations. Now we recognize that people can and do act from unconscious motives. However, many respected theorists still hold to a basically cognitive model and many more incorporate at least some element of cognitive theory into their frameworks.

Hedonism

Hedonism holds that persons act to obtain satisfaction and avoid pain or discomfort. While it is obvious that this forms the motivation for many actions, it does not explain them all; nor does it explain how we can be conditioned to do things that we do not want to do or normally would not do.

Instinct Theories

Instinct theories explain motivation by saying that it is inherent, an identical behavior pattern found in everyone. Although instinct may play a significant part in our lives, much disagreement exists among theoreticians about whether such "instincts" are inborn or learned.

Drive Theories

Drive theories take the position that human beings are motivated by conditions to fulfill desires, needs, or wants. Drives are classified as primary (physiological needs such as food, water, sex, and stimulation) or secondary (learned, as for a particular type of food or stimulation). Most of today's theoreticians incorporate at least some element of drive theory into their frameworks.

Maslow

When we discuss motivational theory, three theorists stand out. Maslow is a familiar name to most of us; Herzberg and McGregor are familiar to many.

Maslow's theory of the hierarchy of needs has found widespread acceptance in recent years. Maslow (1968) postulates that each person is motivated by many specific needs, which fall into general categories and which can be placed on levels from highest to lowest. When a lower need is met, we move on to meet the next highest level.

The most basic level of need is the physiological. Food, drink, shelter, and relief from pain are necessities for everyone. Physiological needs occur independently rather than in combination (Lancaster, 1980, p. 47). These most basic needs are overwhelming until satisfied and must be met before we can progress to satisfy higher levels of needs.

The next level on the hierarchy is safety and security. Both physical and psychological safety are issues. These needs begin to deal with aspects beyond the immediate time frame. The need for protection against threat, both from the environment and from others, and for basic assurances about the future are central.

Next are the needs for love, belonging, and social interaction. Once the basic requirements for physiology and security are met, relationships with others become the focus. The need to be loved and to be productive, fully acknowledged members of groups motivates many of us.

Those levels are followed by the level of autonomy and self-esteem. Once assured that we are loved, and feeling part of a group, we desire to be recognized, valued, and appreciated for ourselves as individuals rather than for what we offer the group.

The highest level is that of self-actualization, the realization of creativity and our fullest potentials as human beings. This level is rarely fully met, as we crave continued self-development and creative outlets.

These needs overlap. The basic requirements for food, shelter, and security remain and must be satisfied on an ongoing basis, but higher level needs become increasingly dominant.

Herzberg

Another well recognized theoretician on the subject of motivation is Frederick Herzberg (1968). Dr. Herzberg postulates that human beings have two opposing sides, which he labels Adam and Abraham. The Adam side is the instinctive, animal side; the Abraham side is the rational, thinking side capable of realizing our full potential.

Herzberg discusses job satisfaction. He postulates that job satisfaction is related to motivators, the most important being achievement, recognition, the work itself, responsibility, and advancement. He labels as hygiene factors those things (company policies and administration, supervision, salary, interpersonal relationships and working conditions) that may serve to prevent job dissatisfaction but that cannot in and of themselves create satisfaction for an individual. The factors involved in job satisfaction are separate and distinct from those that lead to job dissatisfaction.

McGregor

Another theorist we must consider is Douglas McGregor (1960). McGregor synthesized the theories of others into what he called Theory X and Theory Y. Theory X, the traditional approach to work and workers, postulates that workers are inherently lazy and seek to do as little as possible. Managers must therefore direct and control workers if they are to be productive. Theory Y, on the other hand, assumes that people desire to be productive and want to be effective and responsible workers. Managers, therefore, who are proponents of Theory X take a participative, democratic approach to leading others.

None of these theories by themselves is adequate to explain what does or does not motivate individuals. But taken together they provide a framework within which we can begin to understand motivation. Figure 13-1 shows the relationship of Maslow and Herzberg to a motivation situation. The resulting behavior will be influenced by the leadership style of the supervisor.

Motivational Factors

Why cover motivation in a chapter on supervision? Job performance is a result of the interaction between two factors: the ability to perform the job and the motivation to do so. Both are essential for effective performance.

Figure 13-1 The Relationship of Maslow and Herzberg to a Motivation Situation

MASLOW

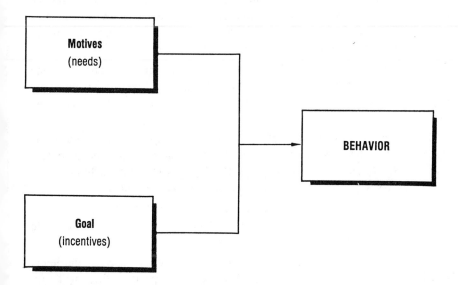

HERZBERG

From *Management of Organizational Behavior: Utilizing Human Resources* (4th ed.) (p. 60) by P. Hersey and K. Blanchard, 1982, Englewood Cliffs, NJ: Prentice-Hall. Copyright © 1982. Reprinted by permission.

It is important to recognize that we cannot really motivate others; we can only modify the climate so that individuals can motivate themselves. Each individual is unique, and therefore different things will be important to each person. The ability to apply these concepts will be needed by both coordinators and preceptors. Both must create a motivating environment in which it is possible to grow and in which individual efforts are recognized and appreciated.

Motivation occasionally becomes a problem for novices or preceptors. An examination of the following factors can be important in diagnosing and intervening appropriately. First, what is the person's individual need for achievement? How does he or she define accomplishment, and how is his or her need for it being met? Each preceptor or novice defines achievement in an individual way. To one person, it will be numbers of patients cared for, to another it will be the quality of care those patients received, to yet another it will be a pat on the back for a special project. What makes the person go home at night feeling good about what he or she did?

Next, look at hygiene factors. Does the individual believe that he or she is well paid for work done? Do company policies seem reasonable and fair? Are relationships with co-workers and supervisors positive? While hygiene factors alone cannot cause job satisfaction, their absence can contribute to dissatisfaction.

Does the job require skills and abilities that are valued and that the individual believes he or she possesses? Motivation decreases if people believe the job they are doing is of insufficient value to the organization or manager or if employees believe they lack the skills necessary to adequately perform the job.

Is adequate feedback given? Expectations for performance must be clear, and individuals must receive sufficient feedback for them to determine if those expectations have been met. Insufficient feedback is often a cause of inadequate performance.

Do the preceptors or novices have an opportunity to participate in decisions that will affect them? While this is not always possible, if staff members feel included it will decrease dissatisfaction. Participation in events, activities, and decisions that will affect one's future can be a strong motivator.

Is performance important to advancement or acceptability? The belief that one's personal performance is irrelevant will strongly reduce motivation to do a good job or to care about one's performance.

Obviously, each individual will have differing needs for each of the items listed above. Some will have strong needs for participation; others will find participation of less importance than personal recognition. But all are important, and an examination of them can be of use in developing the full potential of both novices and preceptors.

Goals

Crucial to motivation is the setting of goals. Goals define intents and allow us to outline processes for personal or professional development. Goals must be mutually set. While they should encompass the recommendations of the coordinator or preceptor, they must not consist exclusively of coordinator or preceptor desires.

Setting goals sounds easy. In reality it is more complicated, as it is easy to become diverted. Goals must meet four criteria: they must be conceivable, believable, measurable, and desirable.

First, goals must be conceivable. It is useless to set a goal of reaching the moon if technology has not yet progressed beyond the horse and buggy. This seems a far-fetched analogy, but novices (and sometimes the rest of us) have been known to set goals far out of reach for ourselves at the moment. We must crawl before we can walk. Too high a goal is discouraging rather than motivating.

Goals must be believable. Participants setting the goals must believe they can be reached. Frequently we hear "I can't do that," and, since the person believes it is so, he or she never will. The reaction to someone else saying "You'll never do that" varies. Sometimes it becomes a self-fulfilling prophecy; at other times it spurs the individual to accomplishments once thought impossible.

Goals must be measurable. How else will you know when the goal has been reached? Again, it sounds simple. But many of us set goals for ourselves ("I will lose weight") without any measurable component. It is impossible to measure progress if we are not moving toward a specific end. In addition, to retain motivation the steps toward the goal must be small enough so that progress is made within a relatively short period of time but not so small as to make achieving them worth nothing to us.

Goals must be desirable. This reminds us that goals are not always set in the direction that we would wish and that, from the coordinator's standpoint, undesirable or unsuitable goals are probably worse than no goals at all.

Once goals are set, the plan to meet those goals must be identified. This plan will vary, depending on the type of goal set and the strengths of the individual. Resources should be identified to assist the individual if that is appropriate. If applicable, consequences of failure to meet the goal (such as termination if a set standard of performance is not reached) should be spelled out.

Hersey and Blanchard (1982) have developed a framework for management that serves well as a model. Their structure is based on how well the follower achieves goals or accomplishes tasks. They describe four levels of mastery, based on the amount of intervention needed by the leader.

Leaders base their interventions on the level of the follower's independence in achieving a particular goal or completing a specific task. The steps are not necessarily incremental, and the same individual may move between the levels depending on the goal or task and the circumstances of the moment.

Telling

The first level is that of telling. Here, the follower is unable and unwilling to meet the goal. The role of the leader is to tell the follower how to accomplish the task and to give appropriate encouragement. This is often the situation that new novices are in when faced with a new procedure or activity. They lack both the know-how and the motivation to proceed. The preceptor therefore will need to clearly instruct them on how to accomplish the activity, to supervise them in doing so, and to provide the support and encouragement needed for them to attempt the task.

Selling

The second level is selling. The follower is willing but lacks the ability to do the job. The manager's role is therefore to assist the novice in gaining the necessary knowledge or skills. Preceptors or coordinators will need to "explain decisions and provide opportunities for clarification" (Hersey & Blanchard, 1982, p. 161). The attitude of "let me help you with that" and of working with the novices to help them gain the requisite information and know-how is central to developing competent individuals.

Participating

The next level is participating. In this situation, the follower is not willing but is able to do the task. Often this is the case with novices; they have the theoretical knowledge but fear putting it into practice. Leaders must therefore use a supportive, nondirective approach ("Let's see what happens when you arrange it this way").

Delegating

The final level is delegation. Individuals at this stage are both willing and able and need little direction or support. A delegative style that permits independence and individual decision making is best when individuals are at this level.

To effectively delegate one must keep several principles in mind. First, be sure that the person you are delegating to is really ready to handle the assignment, that sufficient experience, education, training, and motivation are present and that the individual's judgment is adequate to handle the assignment. It is always best to start with small tasks and build than to delegate too much in the beginning.

Starting small and building allows you to assess the ability of the individual to assume other responsibilities and builds on successes.

Clearly set expectations. Explain what is to be done, by when, and how if appropriate. Be sure the person you are delegating to understands your instructions and is clear about them.

Be available to answer questions, but don't hover. However frustrating it is to need clarification and not be able to get it, it is more disturbing to have a task delegated to you and then have all or part of it done by a nervous preceptor or coordinator or have someone hovering over you while you (nervously) try to carry out the task. Once you are reasonably comfortable that they can do the job, allow novices to do it.

Build authority in. Let others know who will be responsible for the task and direct them to that person when they have questions or need direction. This is especially important in situations such as team leading, when others are used to looking to you for direction and aren't yet trusting of the new individual. Unless novices are expected to make decisions and take responsibility for them during their tenures as novices, they cannot be expected to fully assume the responsibility for decision making later. Arrange checkpoints as appropriate. This helps to assure the novice that he or she is on the right track and provides an opportunity for you to intervene if necessary. Such checkpoints will depend on the activity delegated but might include a daily check-in on how the diabetic teaching is going, for example, a quick runthrough to be sure all equipment is gathered before a procedure, or a review of an evaluation after it is written but before it is given.

Be aware that there is always a risk in delegating. You need to be prepared to deal with unorthodox approaches or wrong decisions. Many of these can be avoided if checkpoints are carefully adhered to, but no such system is foolproof. Be alert to cues that tell you things are not as they should be and be prepared to intervene if conflict arises.

HANDLING CONFLICT

Whenever the topic of supervision surfaces, so does the subject of handling conflict. For some reason, it often seems impossible to have more than one person working without having conflict.

Conflicts arise from a variety of sources. Some of the most common are due to different value systems, competition, unclear or overlapping responsibilities, or disagreements over methods or goals.

Conflicts that are due to differing value systems are among some of the most difficult to handle. The key is to recognize what is happening. Sometimes simply recognizing the source of the conflict by the parties involved is sufficient to decrease or eliminate the conflict. It is important to communicate to all parties that opinions and values are personal, and that they needn't change simply because the other party has difficulty accepting your values. Nevertheless, a mutual means of communicating and a system for working together must be found.

Conflicts that are due to competition are common. Again, recognition of the source of conflict is important but such conflicts are unlikely to cease simply because the source is recognized. A clear statement from the coordinator is important in such instances. Novices should be aware that they are not competing against one another or against staff already in the role they are pursuing but that they are being measured against the criteria outlined in the program plan. A clear understanding of the evaluation criteria and an approach supportive of all novices can help to avert this potential conflict, as can the clear expectation that the novices will support one another rather than competing against one another.

Unclear or overlapping responsibilities can become a source of conflict. This is a common cause of conflict between novices and preceptors as they normally share patient assignments. Clear expectations regarding what each is doing and what each expects of the other and open communication channels can eliminate the problem. When conflict of this type threatens to become a problem, the involved parties need to sit down, clear the air, renegotiate what each is doing, and be sure that both parties have a clear understanding.

Disagreements over methods or goals can also be a source of conflict. Frequently, these conflicts originate in a difference in priorities or values. If one person believes that there is only one correct way to do a procedure and the other believes there are multiple ways, conflict is almost inevitable. Again, open communication and mutual problem solving will usually resolve the problem.

In most instances, compromise or negotiation over what is to be done, when, and how is possible. If conflict continues, however, or a settlement cannot be reached, the coordinator may need to reexamine the preceptor-novice match or reconsider the inclusion of the preceptor.

SUMMARY

In this chapter the topics of leadership and motivation were explored in relation to the responsibilities of supervision. Occasionally, the performance of a preceptor or novice falls below acceptable standards. Giving criticism kindly but effectively is difficult for most of us. Even if performance is exceptional, periodic reviews are necessary. The issues of performance appraisal and evaluation are complex ones for any preceptor or coordinator. The next chapter will be devoted to these topics.

REFERENCES

Hersey, P., & Blanchard, K. (1982). *Management of organizational behavior: Utilizing human resources* (4th ed.). Englewood Cliffs, NJ: Prentice-Hall.

Herzberg, F. (1968) One more time: How do you motivate employees? *Harvard Business Review,* 46(1), 53–62.

Lancaster, J. (1980). *Adult psychiatric nursing.* Garden City, NY: Medical Examination Co.

Maslow, A.H. (1968). *Toward a psychology of being* (2nd ed.). New York: Van Nostrand Reinhold.

McGregor, D. (1960). *The human side of enterprise.* New York: McGraw-Hill.

Murray, J.E. (1964). *Motivation and emotion.* Englewood Cliffs, NJ: Prentice-Hall.

Smoyak, S.A. (1978). Teaching as coaching. *Nursing Outlook,* 26(6), 361–363.

Vroom, V.H., & Yetten, P.W. (1973). *Leadership and decision making.* Pittsburgh: University of Pittsburgh Press.

Washington State Practical Nurse Practice Act. RCW 18.78.

Webster's seventh new collegiate dictionary. (1967). Springfield, MA: G. & C. Merriam.

Chapter 14

Performance Appraisal

Think of the word "evaluation." What thoughts or feelings come to mind? Most preceptors would describe themselves as being nervous, anxious, or fearful. The feelings evoked are usually negative. Few think of words such as "growing," "exciting," "happy."

As few preceptors have written evaluations previously, their feelings are inextricably tied with those they experienced when receiving evaluations. Preceptor feelings about evaluation usually fall into one of three categories: fear, anger, or guilt. Let us look at each of these categories in more depth.

Most preceptors are anxious or fearful. What will they say? How will the novice react? How will they respond to the novice's reaction? Must they justify themselves? How? Can they change, or help others to change? Fear and anxiety result from feelings of inadequacy in dealing with evaluations.

Anger is not uncommon, particularly if it is felt that evaluations might be unfair. An inadequate evaluation tool will frequently provoke anger. Often this anger is directed at the coordinator, who is perceived to be responsible for the evaluation tool or structure. Anger results from a feeling of threat and an attempt to destroy that threat. Preceptors also fear anger in their novices, anticipating difficulty in handling it constructively.

Guilt also occurs. Preceptors sometimes feel that it is their fault that the novice didn't succeed. They ask themselves what more could have been done and often hate criticizing someone else when they themselves are imperfect. Guilt is anger turned inward and it produces depression, feelings of incompetence and powerlessness.

These feelings are common when preceptors discuss either giving or receiving criticism. And it is criticism that is thought of when evaluations are discussed— either having to give or receive them. Yet evaluations can be positive experiences, helping persons to grow as individuals.

WHY HAVE EVALUATIONS?

Evaluations serve several purposes. They provide an appraisal of progress. Without a point at which individuals could force themselves to stand back, look at what they are doing, why, and where they are currently as opposed to where they want to be, many would continue daily tasks without ever pausing. Evaluations provide that needed reminder to stop, reexamine personal or professional lives, and look at exactly what is being done and why. We will never recognize how far we've come if we don't occasionally pause to look back. Likewise, we won't know where we want to go.

Evaluations provide feedback. As essential as feedback is, few persons receive enough during daily routines. When feedback is received, it is usually negative: what was done incorrectly rather than correctly. Evaluation provides a structured time for both positive and negative feedback and forces individuals to either give or listen to that information.

Evaluation is an opportunity for the diagnosis of strengths, a chance to hear what was done correctly. It is an important element in job performance and self-esteem for everyone.

Evaluation also provides a time to assess needs stemming from both the diagnosed strengths and weaknesses and an opportunity to plan to meet those needs. This is a time to sit down together, validate impressions of work performance, and reflect on those areas where improvement is needed. More important, a design to improve can be negotiated, facilitating growth both as employees and as human beings.

GIVING EVALUATIONS

Since preceptors are likely to be in the uncomfortable position of having to write and give evaluations, we'll begin with that and discuss receiving criticism when we discuss how people react to evaluations.

First, be sure that all parties are familiar with the evaluation process. Both preceptors and novices should be aware of the time and number of evaluations, the format, the responsibilities of both parties in the evaluation process, and of the procedure for routing written appraisals.

Before preceptors begin writing an evaluation, or performance appraisals (the terms are synonymous), they need sufficient information to make accurate assessments. Therefore, they must monitor the novice's performance. This means that sufficient observations, under various situations, must be made to get a true feeling of how the novice performs. Basing an evaluation on only one or two observations or incidents is unfair and gives a skewed picture of the individual's overall abilities.

Preceptors should observe all aspects of the job. A preceptor cannot evaluate an individual's patient teaching skills, for example, if he or she has never watched the novice teach a patient. This sounds incredibly basic, but often preceptors tend to generalize. For example, having watched a novice teach another staff person, the preceptor expands that to "That novice is really good at patient teaching." That may be the case, but unless the preceptor has watched the novice with a patient this is not certain.

Help preceptors to examine their biases and subjective judgments. We all have them. If we're aware of them, they are less likely to get in the way of fairness and objectivity. Biases stem from value systems. Values influence everything we do. There are biases that are obvious, such as being pro- or anti-abortion or thinking that all male nurses are gay, and more subtle ones such as thinking that unless one works in an intensive care setting one isn't really competent, or that if all the baths and beds aren't finished by 10 a.m. one isn't a good nurse. It's not wrong to have biases; they simply need to be recognized as such. Preceptors must be careful that they don't unfairly influence evaluations.

The halo effect is a common bias in evaluation. This refers to the tendency of the evaluator to allow a rating in one area to unduly influence ratings in other areas. In other words, to generalize. The rating of an individual as outstanding in initiative, for example, may artificially inflate other aspects of the rating. Preceptors need to be aware of this tendency and try to avoid it as they are evaluating novices.

Be sure to instruct preceptors to document their observations while they are observing. These notes can provide specific examples to illustrate evaluative points and supply the basis for an overall picture of how the novice is doing.

Don't permit preceptors to wait until evaluation time to provide feedback. Feedback should be continuous. Even though this is often difficult as both preceptors and novices become caught up in the activities around them, it is critical. Nothing at the time of the formal evaluation should be new information—it should all have been said before. Evaluations should not be surprise sessions.

Provide assistance and help preceptors to provide assistance to their novices as needed. Again, don't wait until the evaluation conference to share information on the problem or to inform the novice or preceptor of available resources. Work with preceptors from the time that a problem with the novice is discovered. This makes evaluation easier also, as feedback can be provided on the progress made.

In the same vein, help preceptors to acknowledge and reward performance. Periodic mild positives, spaced throughout the program, for example, are stronger than one resounding positive during the evaluation. Don't let preceptors be afraid to tell novices they are doing well and that their progress is noted. This needn't be gushy, but simply an acknowledgment of something done exceptionally well or a quick comment that reinforces the importance or helpfulness of the novice to the preceptor or department.

The Evaluation Conference

The evaluation conference is one of the most nerve-racking events faced by preceptors or novices. If it is well planned and carefully thought out, however, at least some of their anxiety can be reduced.

Have preceptors set a specific time and place for the evaluation conference. "We'll do it sometime this week," or even "We'll do it sometime on Thursday," is vague and tension producing. For the preceptor, opportunities for procrastination are too available and tempting, and for the novice it's like waiting endlessly for the worst to happen. Set a specific time ("after report on Tuesday") and place ("in the conference room") for the evaluation and stick to it.

Have preceptors give the novice time to prepare, and provide specific suggestions for doing so. For example: "We'll meet to go over your evaluation Tuesday after report in the conference room. You might be thinking about one area where you feel you've really improved or that you feel really good about and one goal you like to work on during the next three weeks."

Help preceptors prepare themselves as well. Focus them on what they want to accomplish in the evaluation and develop a plan. If they are anxious about the conference, it may help to write out an opening statement and consider probable responses from the novice in advance. Encourage them to allow sufficient time and to set aside time for discussion. Evaluation should be a two-way conversation, not a one-way lecture.

Set the climate carefully. The environment should be a private one where novice and preceptor won't be continually interrupted. If a private room or space can't be found, encourage preceptors to rearrange their furniture to provide as much privacy as possible. Don't encourage giving an evaluation in the center of a busy nursing station with doctors, staff, and patients interrupting. It isn't possible for either the novice or preceptor to concentrate.

The psychological environment of the evaluation is as important as the physical environment. The atmosphere should be warm, friendly, and relaxed, yet businesslike. Preceptors should not present themselves as detached, cold, or unfeeling; nor should the attitude be a punitive or threatening one. A supportive environment encourages collaborative problem solving.

Encourage preceptors to be direct. New preceptors often find this the most difficult aspect of evaluation. Both novice and preceptor know the reason for the meeting. While a few moments of social niceties can help to break the tension, more is distracting. Concentrate on the issue at hand—the individual's performance.

Stress truthfulness, and not beating around the bush. If there are negatives, address them first. Don't sandwich negatives between two positives; it dilutes the effect of both. Preceptors should be encouraged to be calm, firm, and objective. Sharing their feelings and using "I" statements warm up the interaction and convey a sense of caring. "Joan, I don't feel you are working up to your full potential." "Sarah, I find your continual lateness is disruptive to both the unit and myself." Encourage specificity. Being vague or wishy-washy just makes things worse, as does being apologetic about the criticism. Preceptors have both the right and responsibility to demand good performance and apologizing or making excuses weakens the case for it.

If self-evaluation forms are being used, try having the novice give the preceptor his or her self-evaluation first. This provides a jumping off point for mutual discussion and allows comment on the novice's assessment of skills and abilities rather than the preceptor starting out cold. Often the novice's self-evaluation will be far harsher then the preceptor's assessment and the preceptor can provide reassurance and support instead of criticism—a far more comfortable situation for the new preceptor.

Constructive Feedback

Confronting someone with a marginal or unacceptable performance is difficult. The following rules can help preceptors give constructive feedback if they must correct or admonish novices' performance.

First, make sure that the issue is important. Don't bother with trivialities. There is no point in wasting your time if the matter is inconsequential or immaterial. In addition, it must be possible for the individual to change. There is no point in chastizing someone who does not have the capacity to improve.

Pick times carefully. Discussions should occur as soon after the event as possible. Lapses of time between the correction and the event tend to diminish its importance.

Don't give criticism at the end of the day or Friday afternoons. This may seem to conflict with the second rule, but it really doesn't. Address the issue as quickly after the act as possible but do it at a time when it will be received in the best manner. At the end of the day or the week generally isn't the best time. The person being criticized is tired, will have difficulty focusing, and will go home and worry about it. Things are always worse when we're alone or have undivided time to mull over a reprimand. Preceptors need to have the time, during the remainder of the day or week to reassure the novice with their tone of voice, words, and attitude, convincing the novice that it is the act not the person with which there is discontent.

Keep it private. What has to be said should be a confidential matter between the preceptor and the novice. Never criticize in public. To do so is a show of power, and is counterproductive. In the long run power will be lost, because respect will be lost.

Give the novice undivided attention. Arrange not to be interrupted; have phone calls answered by someone else. Concentrate on the interaction and don't become distracted.

Be specific and direct. Give the facts and don't be ambiguous. Use examples from your observations. Avoid using "always" and "never"; they are vague terms and imply superficiality you would do best to avoid.

Take one issue at a time. Otherwise, continuity may be lost by skipping back and forth. Don't unload all frustrations and problems in one setting. Overloading accomplishes nothing. More will be gained if the important issues are addressed first and the less important ones later on.

Face the facts squarely. Don't use vague references or subtle euphemisms to talk about specific performance deficiencies. Don't sandwich praise between criticism or vice versa. This dilutes the effect of both. Give the criticism, then the praise. Giving the weakness first emphasizes its importance. Giving the praise later helps begin the healing process and tells the individual that there are things that he or she does well.

Redirect and refocus the conversation if needed. Many persons being told of inadequate work react with hostility. There is often an attempt to justify or sidestep the issue or to avoid dealing directly with the matter. You must retain the focus on the behavior change desired by redirecting the conversation:

—"I forgot. . ." "What can be done to be sure it won't happen again? What can we do to help you remember?"

—"I'm sorry. . ." "How can you avoid having it happen again?"

—"No one told me." "Now that you know, what can you do?"

—"It's not my fault; it's someone else's." "Maybe, but what can you do to help?"

—"Ok, Ok, I'll try to do better." (No definite solution) "I appreciate that. What specifically will you do?"

Criticize the act, not the person. You dislike the act, not the person. An example: the preceptor who says to a novice "You were really stupid yesterday" rather than discussing the specific acts that were a problem. Describe the unacceptable behavior, not personality characteristics. Personal characteristics are important only as they contribute to performance.

Criticize without comparison. Don't have favorites. Comparing is unfair. Everyone has areas of strength and weakness. Having someone else's strengths paraded in front of one doesn't help; it causes anger and resentfulness.

Be serious. If the behavior is serious enough to warrant criticism, it deserves to be treated as such. A frivolous or lighthearted approach is inappropriate.

Don't expect to win a popularity contest. Novices sometimes criticize preceptors. Encourage the preceptor to take ownership of the situation and not to make excuses or apologize. Precepting performance is irrelevant. Although it is difficult to ignore comments such as "If you were a better preceptor I wouldn't have this problem," help preceptors not to focus on the novice's criticism for the moment. The preceptor's job is to be sure that the performance is corrected, not to be sure that he or she is liked. As coordinator, you will have to help preceptors to accept and put this into practice.

Finally, don't just discuss the complaint, even if specifically. Ask for a reasonable change to relieve the problem. Identify the remedy as specifically as the error. Use open-ended questions to explore and stimulate thinking. "How are you going to solve this problem?" Let the novice come up with the solution. Preceptors may suggest alternatives but should be encouraged to allow novices to choose the solutions they would like to try. Preceptors should voice their expectations specifically. "I expect from now on . . ." At the end of the conversation, there should be a specific plan for what will be done to correct the matter. Appendix J contains exercises for giving criticism constructively and specifically.

Setting Goals

Once the discussion of performance is completed, set future goals. These should include a clear description of the desired change, the process to use (if applicable), when it must be done by, and how you will know it's done. The final summing up of the goal might be "Joan, I expect to see an improvement in the areas we discussed within the next three weeks." "Sarah, I expect you to be on time from now on."

At the end of the conference, sum up what was decided and reaffirm your expectations. Both participants should be clear on the behavior change desired and the actions that will be taken.

FOLLOWTHROUGH

Be prepared to help the preceptor follow through. Urge preceptors to reward the novice for improved performance, and let them know that the improvement has been noticed. When progress is made, both the novice and the preceptor will feel good.

What does the preceptor do if performance doesn't improve or if it doesn't improve adequately? What if the plan was abandoned or never carried to completion? Or if after several more coaching and counseling sessions there still isn't adequate progress?

Although the cooperation and support of the preceptor is still essential, this is usually the point at which the coordinator must assume active responsibility for dealing with the problem. Often the coordinator's active involvement and intervention is sufficient. If not, further interventions must be planned.

There are no real rules to follow, but there are alternatives. In any given situation there are three choices: accept the situation and learn to live with it, change it, or get out.

In some situations, living with it may be the best alternative. If the individual's performance is such that you can live with the deficiency, then you may choose to do so. Be aware, however, that the price may be more than you are really willing to pay. Retaining someone whose performance is marginal may have a demoralizing effect on the remainder of the department and can cause resentment, hostility, and indignation from other staff.

You have already tried to change the situation and have failed. Unless you can come up with other ideas to try, this choice is out.

Getting out is the final choice. This may mean that you get out, but more likely it means getting the marginal performer out. This may take one of two formats: transfer or termination.

Often a transfer is a viable solution and works out well for everyone concerned. If a position is available that better fits the strengths and requires less of the weaknesses, the "problem" employee may bloom in a different position. Be alert, however, to the assumption by others that you are trying to dump your problem onto them. Assess the climate before you arrange to move someone.

The final solution is to terminate someone. There are instances where this is the best alternative for everyone, including the employee. If things have reached such an impasse that, even if the employee turned into the best novice ever, the situation couldn't be turned around, it is best to terminate. Failure to act responsibly can only hurt both the individual and the organization. Be sure that you have discussed the matter with your personnel department and that institutional, departmental, and program policies for disciplinary action, probation, suspension, and termination have been followed.

HANDLING CRITICISM

Regardless of how well you handle evaluations, it is likely that preceptors will be criticized by someone. No matter how competent we are, someone always disagrees with what we do or how we do it. However, criticism doesn't have to destroy self-esteem.

When preceptors begin to worry about what was said, they often find themselves mentally playing mistakes over and over in their heads. "Yeah, she's right. I can't do anything right. I always goof it up. Just like I did last week. And last Tuesday." Thinking of the negative experiences causes them to think of more negatives. Soon they can't remember any positives.

It is usually not the comment but the emotional switch it triggers that turns on "negative tapes." People tend to react to criticism in one of three ways: the "I'm no good" reaction (replaying past mistakes), the "You're no good" reaction (playing feelings about the person criticizing), or the "I'll learn from this" reaction (reaffirming self-esteem). These three reactions and common thinking distortions are depicted in Exhibits 14-1 and 14-2.

Exhibit 14-1 Coping with Criticism

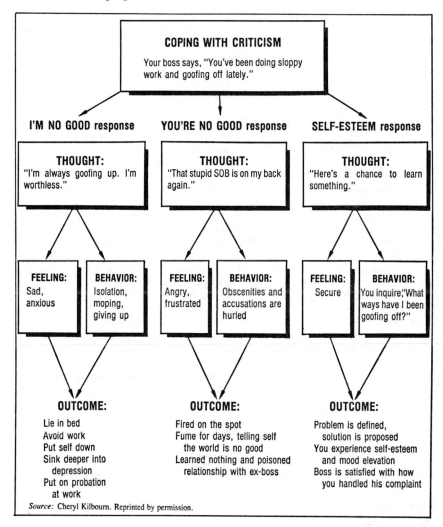

The "I'm no good" and "You're no good" reactions result from disturbances in self-esteem. The "I'm no good" reaction plays negative tapes. This response puts oneself down. Mentally, the situation is retreated from and hurt and anxiety are turned on. Automatic credence is given to the person criticizing. The "You're no good" reaction also stems from poor self-esteem but anger, disappointment, or hurt are turned outward and the person who criticizes is attacked.

The self-esteem response is the most productive one. It approaches the situation as one that can be learned from. With an open mind that neither automatically

Exhibit 14-2 Definitions of Cognitive Distortions

1. **ALL-OR-NOTHING THINKING:** You see things in black and white categories. If your performance falls short of perfect, you see yourself as a total failure.
2. **OVERGENERALIZATION:** You see a single negative event as a never-ending pattern of defeat.
3. **MENTAL FILTER:** You pick out a single negative detail and dwell on it exclusively so that your vision of all reality becomes darkened, like the drop of ink that discolors the entire beaker of water.
4. **DISQUALIFYING THE POSITIVE:** You reject positive experiences by insisting they "don't count" for some reason or other. In this way you can maintain a negative belief that is contradicted by your everyday experiences.
5. **JUMPING TO CONCLUSIONS:** You make a negative interpretation even though there are no definite facts that convincingly support your conclusion.
  a. Mind reading. You arbitrarily conclude that someone is reacting negatively to you, and you don't bother to check this out.
  b. The Fortune Teller Error. You anticipate that things will turn out badly, and you feel convinced that your prediction is an already-established fact.
6. **MAGNIFICATION (CATASTROPHIZING) OR MINIMIZATION:** You exaggerate the importance of things (such as your goof-up or someone else's achievement), or you inappropriately shrink things until they appear tiny (your own desirable qualities or the other fellow's imperfections). This is also called the "binocular trick."
7. **EMOTIONAL REASONING:** You assume that your negative emotions necessarily reflect the way things really are: "I feel it, therefore it must be true."
8. **SHOULD STATEMENTS:** You try to motivate yourself with shoulds and shouldn'ts, as if you had to be whipped and punished before you could be expected to do anything. "Musts" and "oughts" are also offenders. The emotional consequence is guilt. When you direct such statements toward others, you feel anger, frustration, and resentment.
9. **LABELING AND MISLABELING:** Extreme form of overgeneralization. Instead of describing error, you attach negative label to self: "I'm a loser." Or negative label to someone else: "He's a louse." Highly colored language and emotionally loaded.
10. **PERSONALIZATION:** You see yourself as the cause of some negative external event which in fact you were not primarily responsible for.

Source: Cheryl Kilbourn. Reprinted by permission.

believes nor disbelieves what has been said, an attempt to gain more information and self-knowledge is made.

Just as one learns to handle compliments gracefully, preceptors can learn to handle criticism. They first need to learn how to handle themselves and form a framework to work from when criticized. Through practice, they can then learn to handle themselves appropriately when they feel attacked.

The framework consists of three steps: active listening, promoting verbalization, and problem solving. First, use active listening to calm the critic. Avoid being defensive or judgmental. A first reaction when attacked is often to retaliate with something like "Oh yeah, well, your charting isn't so good either." This serves no purpose and only alienates others. Don't worry about the individual's motive in criticizing you. It really doesn't matter at this point.

Use empathy. Try to see the world through the other person's eyes. Use feelings ("I feel" or "You feel") statements instead of thinking ("I think" or "You think") statements. Criticism deals with feelings and emotions, not with thoughts and beliefs. Don't correct a statement of feelings. You cannot tell others what they should or should not feel.

Find out the specifics. How was the individual offended? What was done? When? How often does it happen? What else is bothering this person about the situation? The purpose of probing for such information is not to receive a catalogue of all that is done wrong but to clear the air and establish a starting point to talk from. Often the feelings have built up over a period of time and must be expressed before constructive conversation can begin.

Find something you can agree with. This disarms the critic. If the criticism is justified, agree with it. "You're right. I haven't been getting to work on time lately." If you feel it isn't justified, find something in what the person says with which you can agree: "I'm sorry you feel that way." That's true. You are sorry this person feels that way. You don't agree but you are sorry. Be truthful and sincere.

Encourage verbalization. Again, try to "get it all out." Let the person wind down before you try to deal with the specifics of what was said. Affirming the person's anger acknowledges that it was heard and that there is a willingness to respond. Disallowing anger heightens it.

Once you have gone through these two steps, you are ready to move on to the specific situation. Whether deciding to confront the individual, ignore the criticism, or debate it, remain responsive and sincere. An attitude of caring will make the difference between a productive session that leaves both parties feeling better or an unproductive, hostile encounter.

SUMMARY

This chapter has discussed giving performance appraisals, especially giving criticism. We have focused on making evaluations a productive and less stressful experience. The next chapter will focus on preceptor self-care.

Chapter 15

Preceptor Self-Care

This chapter introduces the idea of preceptor self-care: the management of stress, time, and burnout for preceptors.

Why are we talking about such things? After all, precepting is supposed to be rewarding, a way to recognize individual nurses for their talents and skills. Unfortunately, preceptors may need such help far more than others in the organization.

Nursing is inherently stressful. There are too many things to do in too short a period of time, and there is the added burden of knowing that an error in judgment or technique may prove at best harmful and at worst fatal to another human being. Add to this difficult hours, grumbling doctors, querulous patients, and clamorous families and you have a situation ripe for stress. Add a novice to this scenario and you add one additional thing to do and one additional person to be responsible for in a job where there are already too many things to do and too many persons to be responsible for. Precepting increases the stress of an already stressful job.

For these reasons it is essential to give preceptors the skills needed to deal with the demands they face. Stress and time management are as important for preceptors as for the chief executive officer, if not more so. At least the CEO probably has a secretary to help him or her stay organized.

In addition, preceptors must help their novices to efficiently and effectively use *their* time. Most novices will need considerable help in determining priorities and methods for organization. What previously sounded easy proves more difficult in real life. Therefore, preceptors need assistance in identifying methods with which they can help their novices.

MANAGING TIME

What are the "realities" of time? Despite all wishful thinking and pipe dreams, we have only twenty-four hours a day. No one has more or less. When you think of it, time is the only natural resource that has been distributed perfectly evenly. No matter how rich or how poor, fat or thin, or what job we hold, we have all been blessed with exactly the same twenty-four hours a day. In this finite amount of time we must work, eat, sleep, learn, relax, and commune with others.

For this reason, it behooves all of us to manage our time well. The following, from an unknown author, puts it well:

> This is the beginning of a new day. God has given me this day to use as I will. I can waste it or grow in its light and be of service to others. But what I do with this day is important because I have exchanged a day of my life for it. When tomorrow comes, today will be gone forever. I hope I will not regret the price I paid for it.

To manage time well, we must be both efficient and effective. Efficiency means doing something right the first time. Effectiveness means doing the right thing right (LeBoeuf, 1979).

Planning

Managing time means having control of it. Control starts with planning. Often nurses ask how they can effectively plan their time. They say they have little control over it. Patients and emergencies cause constant interruptions.

To some extent this is true. Both patients and emergencies do provide interruptions. However, that fact demands that we plan our time even more effectively if the things that are important are to be completed and time is not wasted in trivial activities.

How can one effectively plan one's time in nursing? Lakein (1973), and many others, suggests the A, B, C method of priority setting. While this works nicely for paper pushing, it does not seem particularly useful for clinical practice. Everything always seemed to be an A, or at least a B! The plan outlined by Predd (1982) seems to offer a better approach for clinical practice. Predd suggests asking yourself four questions to help plan your days and delegate effectively if the need arises. These are:

1. What must be done immediately?
2. What must be done on a schedule?
3. What must be done sometime during the shift?
4. What would you do if you had the time to do it?

Exhibit 15-1 gives you a practical example of this nursing "To Do" list.

In addition, effective planning requires that we take the time to plan for ourselves. Setting clear goals rather than vague, immeasurable, or idealistic ones

Exhibit 15-1 Nursing "To Do List"

NURSING "TO DO" LIST

Do immediately: ✓ IV's : 440, 42, 43, 45

✓ Breath sounds and chest tubes — Mr. Johnson

Do on schedule:

8ᴬ	Dressing (Mr. Smith) Change IV — Mrs. Pauls (445)
9ᴬ	Meds 40, 41, 43, 44
10ᴬ	Dressing (Mr. Brown)
1030	Conference on Ms. Green
1100	Change IV in 442 ; pre-ops for Ms. Pauls
1200	Check chest tube and breath sounds — Mr. Johnson
100	Meds — 40, 41, 43, 44
200	Change IV — Pauls (Get bottle from pharmacy)
300	Report, change IV in 42

Do sometime: Diabetic teaching Ms. Jones

Ambulate Mr. Smith

Do if time: Call Soc Services to check on Nursing home for Ms. Green

Call Ms. Jones' granddaughter

Shampoo — Jones

From "Setting Priorities: How To Stay Efficient in Hectic Nursing Stations" by C.S. Predd. 1982. *Nursing Life.* 2(3), 50–51. Copyright 1982 by C.S. Predd. Adapted by permission.

can help. This may be a major or long-term goal, such as developing expertise in lecturing, or as small a goal as getting the papers with which to do an evaluation sometime during the shift.

Try "Swiss cheesing" your tasks. This means doing a small amount of a large task at a time; punching holes in it until eventually it is complete. For example, take the evaluation mentioned above. Looked at as one job, the task may seem monumental to fit into a busy daily schedule. Where will you ever find the several hours it will take you to complete the job (without taking it home)?

Let's see what happens when the Swiss cheese approach is used and various pieces are planned into a staff nurse's daily routine. The evaluation is broken out into the following subtasks:

Monday: Get papers.
Tuesday: Review papers; think about what you want to say.
Wednesday: Begin draft of evaluation.
Thursday: Finish draft.
Friday: Edit the evaluation.

In one week the job will have been completed. The various tasks are added to the daily "To Do" list, probably under the "Sometime" section, and both a plan of action and a practical time frame for completing the evaluation, on schedule, and on work time, is formed. Without planning ahead, the evaluation would probably be done the evening before it was due, on the nurse's own time, and without adequately thinking through what to say and how to say it.

Planning ultimately saves time. It gives one a feeling of power and control over what is happening, allows safe and effective delegation of activities to others if the need arises, and demonstrates organization for others (novices). Everyone benefits when the value of planning is acknowledged and time is taken to do it effectively.

How can we combat the failure to plan? For one, the importance of planning must be recognized. Few of us would attempt to build a house without a blueprint, yet we spend much of our lives without clearly knowing where we are going or what the most important things to do along the way are. Once we have recognized the need for and importance of planning we will be much farther along on our way to both efficiency and effectiveness.

Once the importance of planning has been recognized and we have become skilled at doing so, its importance must be conveyed to others. Frequently, especially in nursing, taking a few minutes at the beginning of the shift to plan and organize oneself is seen as wasting time. We need to be able to say (and demonstrate) to others that planning enables us to function more efficiently and effectively, that the time "wasted" saves time later. Results must be stressed rather than the activity.

Haste

Haste is another major time waster. In the rush to get everything done, time is misused. Needing to review things to be sure they are done and done correctly becomes necessary, and things must be done over because due to haste they were not done accurately in the first place.

Combating a compulsion to hurry is essential. If total attention is given to the task at hand each time, the frustration, annoyance, necessity, and time of doing things over is saved. Set realistic time estimates for tasks, procedures, and projects, and recognize that tasks that have never been done will take longer. Proficiency is gained with practice. Complete items the first time. This is analogous to the old rule about handling each piece of paper only once. Get all the data needed before sitting down to write the report or call the physician. This helps you become more organized, presents a more professional picture to others, and saves you time since you need not bounce up and down to retrieve missing information or delay momentum until you can track down the missing pieces.

Crises

Crisis orientations are another time waster. Although obviously in nursing we must be prepared for crises, not everything is a crisis. Distinguish between the urgent and the important, and accomplish the urgent first. Setting priorities is, for nurses, a necessity. Part of setting those priorities is distinguishing for yourself what is urgent to accomplish during the day or week and what is not.

Interruptions

Allow for interruptions. This is a hard lesson for nurses to learn, as their days are a series of constant interruptions. However, we can learn to leave time for those events. MacKensie (1973) suggests that you leave 20 percent of your day for interruptions. For an eight-hour shift, this works out to one and a half hours! Of course, this is not to suggest that any nurse has an hour and a half that can be left totally open, but remember that not all time must be in one lump. Examine your "To Do" list and leave time open where you can. Try to accomplish some of the "sometime" and "like to do" tasks early in the day if possible. This leaves time free to handle the crisis when it arises or, for preceptors, time to teach the novice about the new tube just inserted in the gentleman down the hall. While emergencies probably will disrupt your day, the damage is minimized if the time they take is anticipated.

The "chatter" is also a time waster. Of course, in some cases, this person is trying to tell you something—the wife of the MI patient, in her chatter about her family and sons away in college, is giving you messages that she is worried about her husband and that she doesn't have the support of her family at her side. It is wise to spend the time and allay her anxiety. If you have left discretionary time in the day, this type of interruption will not disrupt your entire day. The social chatter, however, continually interrupts your work to socialize. We have all known persons like this, and most of us have found our own ways to discourage them.

To minimize the chatter's interruptions, you must take control of the situation. When the individual comes to interrupt, ask if it can wait—you are busy right now. Suggest a good time for a chat—perhaps on break or at lunch. Not sitting down is another good technique, as is continuing to edge toward wherever you were going in the first place. To free yourself of the chatter, you must take control of what is happening through your words and body language.

Paperwork

Paperwork is the bane of most nurses' existence, as it keeps us from patients and seems endless. A few suggestions, while not eliminating paperwork altogether, can help to keep it from taking more time than necessary.

First, organize your workspace. Nothing is more frustrating than needing a paper clip and not being able to find one. Or never having a red pen for those entries that require one. Or always having to get another charting form from across the hall. Stop for a moment and look at your workspace. What can you do to make it work better for you? An extra drawer, a box for pens, an additional supply cabinet are probably minor expenses for the unit but may make a tremendous difference in how you are able to operate. Don't just accept the status quo without trying to suggest a change for the better. In addition, keep your work area neat and clean. Organization saves you time.

Use all the tools available to eliminate or minimize paperwork. For example, using flow sheets can help to clearly and concisely document objective data. The data can then be summarized or the note cross-referenced to the flow sheet. However, we often feel the need to completely restate all data documented on the flow sheet or keep similar information in two different files. This duplication is a tremendous waster of our time and adds completely unnecessary steps. Don't do double work.

Pace your paperwork. Charting can be done throughout the day—it needn't wait until 2:30, for example. Evaluations can be spaced throughout the month or year, not all done the same week. If you do pace your paperwork, and the unexpected occurs, you are ahead. If at least some of it hasn't been done, you're looking at another day when you won't be leaving on time because your paperwork isn't done. Try to plan 15 uninterrupted minutes during the day and have someone cover for you. Begin what paperwork you can at that time. Then return the favor for the other person. Ultimately both of you will benefit.

Try "closing the door" and working undisturbed. Frequently, especially in centralized setups, charting time becomes a general coffee klatsch as everyone tries to chart in the same location at the same time. Find an undisturbed (or at least less disturbed) location in which to do your paperwork. This will allow better concentration and ultimately saves time.

Delegate where possible. Perhaps the unit secretary can obtain the evaluation form you need or the nursing assistant take Mrs. Jones that glass of juice. We have a tendency to get trapped into thinking we have to do everything ourselves. Of course, you can't (and don't want to) delegate everything, but ask yourself what is the best use of your time right now? (Lakein, 1973) If your time could best be spent by getting Mr. Smith's medications or doing an evaluation, who else could be getting Mrs. Jones' juice?

The Telephone

Nurses spend a tremendous amount of time on the telephone, but we frequently spend it on hold or waiting for people. This time needn't be wasted. Combine tasks where possible. Begin your charting or an evaluation while waiting for or on the phone, for example. Take a moment to review your "To Do" list and cross out things you have completed while on hold. All too often we waste a few minutes that could have been put to work.

Here are some further tips on phone handling. Have all reference materials handy. Avoid the frustration, for both yourself and the person on the other end of the line, of having to stop while you frantically scramble to find the necessary information. You save yourself both time and aggravation if all reference material (chart, lab work, vital signs, etc.) is at hand.

Have a list of things to cover. It is most exasperating to finish your conversation, hang up, and then realize there was one more question you needed to ask. When you have a list at your fingertips, you can easily scan it while you are finishing your conversation to be sure you have covered all the bases. This saves you and the other party the time and trouble of repeating the call.

If you have an opportunity to leave a message, do so. Give your name, phone number, reason you called, and a time to call you back. This saves you the time of repeatedly calling back only to find that your party has just left, is out on call, or is on another line.

Have someone screen your calls where possible. For example, the ward secretary can find out who the caller is, and if it is not urgent, can take a message and tell the caller you will return the call. This allows you to finish your work and return calls at your convenience. If secretaries are knowledgeable, they can probably answer many of the routine questions, saving you the interruption and the caller the time of waiting. By including unit secretaries in morning report, for example, they often gain sufficient information to answer many of the usual questions from family members and physicians that previously required a nurse. The asking party appreciates not being shuffled from party to party and does not get the feeling that no one knows what is going on. For complicated concerns or more information the asking party is, of course, referred to the nurse or manager.

MANAGING STRESS

Time management is only one aspect of self-care. No discussion of preceptor self-care would be complete without an examination of stress and stress management. What is stress? Although there are many individual definitions, all describe one idea: stress is the body's protective reaction to a real or perceived threat. The threat may be to one's physical, psychological, or social being. Stress causes changes in the feelings, behavior, and physiology of the affected individual.

While we think of stress as primarily negative, it is, in fact, neutral. Stressors, the precipitating factors of stress, may be either positive or negative. For example, working with an extremely bright novice, while rewarding and exciting for the preceptor, may prove extremely stressful as the preceptor tries to find ways to challenge such a learner. Stressors are not identical to emotional arousal or nervous tension since they can occur during anaesthesia or (experimentally) after all neurogenic input is stopped by severing the hypothalmic connections (Selye, 1976, p. 14).

Stress is both a help to survival and a hindrance. Originally, the caveman had to either fight or flee the saber-toothed tiger causing his stress. This released the tensions built up, and he relaxed or, being dead, no longer had to worry about dealing with stress. Modern men and women have more difficulty in dealing with the stressors in their lives, as they cannot, in most cases, either fight or flee from more modern predators.

Physiology

Stress causes specific behavioral, physiological, and psychological changes. Much of the work on physiological reactions to stress has been done by Hans Selye. Dr. Selye became interested in the "syndrome of being sick" while a second-year medical student in Prague, but it was not until he was working in the biochemistry department at McGill University trying to find a new hormone that he began to connect three phenomena, adrenal enlargement, thymiocolympymatic atrophy, and acute gastrointestinal ulcers, into what would eventually become known as the "general adaptation syndrome." This syndrome is based on the theory that the body responds'to stress of any kind with a unified defense mechanism characterized by specific structural and chemical changes. The general adaptation syndrome has three stages.

The first is the stage of alarm, further divided into shock and countershock, where defense mechanisms are mobilized. "We consider the first stage to be the expression of a general alarm of the organism when suddenly confronted with a critical situation" (Selye, 1976, p. 9). During this stage the person undergoes catabolic and other changes that result from the effects of the injury and the response of the body to it. During countershock the individual is restored to his or her preinjury condition.

During the stage of resistance, where full adaptation to the stressor occurs, balance is restored and the person can tolerate greater exposure to the stressor than he or she could in the nonadapted state. If the stressor is strong enough or lasts long enough, the stage of exhaustion inevitably follows since adaptation energy is finite. This stage resembles shock but the ability to adapt is lost and death ensues. The stages are not inviolate; death may occur during the first stage if the stressor is strong enough.

Causes

Stress is caused by numerous factors. Physiological, emotional, intellectual, and other causes are frequent stressors for nurses.

Our normal physical environments abound in stress producers. Noise pollution, air pollution, modern modes of transportation, fashion trends, florescent lights, uncomfortable seating, even gravity cause us effort and energy in dealing with our physical environments.

Social environments are also producers of stress. Families, friends, co-workers, patients, families, and physicians all make never-ending demands on limited amounts of time and stretch the preceptors' limited amounts of resources. Rivalry, jealousy, competition, conflicts in values and acceptable behaviors, concerns over finances, politics, and religious differences cause ongoing tension.

Biology itself causes both physiological and psychological stress. Preceptors and novices alike must respond to physiological, psychological, and developmental stages. Each stage of life has its own particular demands, strains, and resultant stresses. Middle life, as one begins to deal with physical aging, can be equally as stressful as the emotional turbulance of adolescence or the career establishment of the early twenties. Periodic illnesses and injuries add their burden as well.

Nursing itself causes stress. Particularly in the helping professions, idealism and the motivations for entering the profession may become lost in the morass of day-to-day existence within the profession. Altruistic motives become buried as one faces the inept physician, uncaring nurse, overzealous bureaucrat. Conflicts over values and beliefs challenge us daily. The patient wants to die in peace and dignity; modern medicine demands that we do everything we can to prolong life. It is the nurse who is with both the patient and the family and who must help both to make some of the necessary decisions and transitions. Yet nurses themselves receive little support or nurturing. Emotional stresses are constant. Anger, frustration, irritation, negative thinking, and ambivalence are daily companions in modern lives. Preceptors, who must add support and explanations to novices at the same time, live even more stressful existences.

Effects

Like most stresses, a majority of the time these affect us little in our daily lives. Yet they constantly take their toll, and preceptors may suddenly find themselves feeling "stressed out" without really knowing why.

Stress expresses itself in a variety of ways. Just as stress is caused by physiological, emotional, and social factors it manifests itself in these ways.

Physiological symptoms of stress are among its earliest cues. Fatigue, sleep disturbances, sexual difficulties, headaches, muscle aches, indigestion, menstrual distress, anorexia, diarrhea, constipation, palpitations, allergy or asthma attacks, frequent minor illnesses, and a dependence on alcohol or drugs are among the symptoms of unrelieved stress.

Psychosocial symptoms are just as common. Constant feelings of tension; feeling unable to slow down, always feeling pushed, with everything, major and minor, screaming at you to get it done; being unable to focus your attention on the really important things; and a constant feeling of being irritated with everyone and everything are symptoms of unrelieved stress.

Reduction Techniques

Coordinators can help preceptors and novices by increasing their awareness of stressors and by reinforcing the use of stress reduction techniques. An active role, assisting preceptors to recognize and deal with both their own and novices' stress, is essential. Often the signals are minimized or ignored by preceptors, in a belief that they are just part of everyday life or something we can do nothing about.

Help preceptors and novices to be aware of stress both in their lives and their bodies. Be alert to its cues. Help individuals to know what demands cause them stress. Not all persons find the same things stressful—one person may thrive on crowded parties, the next person may find them almost unbearable and must try to avoid or minimize those encounters. Identify those stressors that can be avoided or modified or those that are created by oneself. Frequently we contribute to our stress by putting ourselves in situations we know to be stressful. Help preceptors to set realistic goals for themselves and not to try to accomplish everything at once.

Once it has been recognized, how does one go about reducing stress? Actually, just recognizing stress is a big step forward. A variety of strategies can help preceptors and novices to deal with it. Stress is increased when one feels out of control and powerless. Have a plan for combating your stress. A plan gives direction and a path to follow. Without one you drift aimlessly.

Help preceptors to strive for a balanced lifestyle. Often when we are stressed, perspective is lost and all energies are spent in a single direction. A healthy mixture of work, fun, and leisure will help to balance things.

Develop a repertoire of stress reduction techniques. Relaxation techniques, guided imagery, meditation, and physical activity are some of the measures that have been used successfully to combat stress. Choose those that appeal or have been successful for you and teach or practice them.

Small successes can also help to break the stress rut. Use minor things such as creating a break between work and home by changing clothes, for example. This gives the illusion of breaking one activity from another and will help you to make the mental break.

Coordinators may need to plan periodic breaks for preceptors. Often preceptors are reluctant to admit that they feel they need a break even when they realize it. A sensitivity to overload will assist preceptors to maintain balance and prevent additional stress.

Encourage preceptors and novices to take minibreaks during work. Even a quick, deep breath, combing of the hair, or a stretch can help to combat the daily grind. If possible, a quick breath outside in the fresh air or a fast walk around the block will help. Such a change in activities and pace will refresh and relax. If such strategies are not practiced periodically, stress will eventually lead to burnout.

Burnout

What can be done to avoid the seeming epidemic proportions of burnout among nurses these days?

Burnout is stress out of control (Sanders, 1980), a response to continuous work-related stress (Patrick, 1979). The classic burnout is the reality shock of new graduates so ably described by Kramer (1974). Storlie (1979) describes burnout as a resignation to a lack of power.

McElroy (1982) describes five stages of burnout. During the first stage, physical symptoms predominate. Headaches, frequent colds and flu attacks, fatigue, sleep disturbances, and low energy states are common.

As the stress continues, behavioral or social symptoms appear. Individuals become increasingly unsocial and isolate themselves from the social life going on around them.

Still further along the burnout scale are mental and intelligence disturbances. Individuals find themselves having greater difficulty making decisions and problem-solving ability is impaired. Defensive behavior increases and flexibility decreases.

Ultimately, individuals find themselves almost totally detached from those around them. They have a sense of being personally devalued and begin to devalue others. Cynical behavior increases.

Finally, individuals suffer from an overwhelming sense of guilt. They know they should care but find themselves unable to. Most will leave the occupation or profession. Others remain, but as dehumanized shadows of what they were upon entering the profession.

Burnout can be either system generated or self generated (Patrick, 1979). We generate burnout for ourselves when we demand too much of ourselves. Personal life stresses, such as marital difficulties or financial pressures, combined with emotionally demanding jobs and a lack of self-awareness can easily escalate minor stresses into full-blown burnout syndromes. In addition, self-imposed restrictions on receiving support contribute to feelings of being overwhelmed and an increasing inability to deal with everyday stresses.

Our systems also impose burnout. The sometimes impossible demands of work, coupled with atmospheres that lack nurturance and support systems, increase feelings of isolation and contribute to furtherance of the syndrome. Ultimately, when the individual is mentally and physically exhausted, emotions shift to the negative and feelings of personal and professional devaluation are experienced. By this time one is well into the cycle of burnout.

What can be done about burnout? Here again, recognition is an important step in effective intervention. During initial stages, an increased self-awareness and taking care of oneself can do much to negate the effects of burnout. Exercise, eating well, and getting enough sleep will help to combat continuing stress.

Clarifying values, by deciding what is important, increasing time spent with those persons significant in one's life, finding nurturing relationships both at home and at work, and incorporating adequate time alone will also help to combat stress and prevent burnout.

SUMMARY

This chapter has covered the basics of preceptor self-care, examining time and stress management and the prevention of burnout. Although we end our discussions here, this cannot be the end, for "Whoever acquires knowledge and

does not practice it resembles him who ploughs his land and leaves it unsown''
(Sa'di, 1258/1970).

REFERENCES

Kramer, M. (1974). *Reality shock: Why nurses leave nursing.* St. Louis: Mosby.

Lakein, A. (1973). *How to get control of your time and your life.* New York: New American Library.

LeBoeuf, M. (1979). *Working smart: How to accomplish more in half the time.* New York: McGraw-Hill.

McElroy, A.M. (1982). Burnout—A review of the literature with application to cancer nursing. *Cancer Nursing, 5*(3), 211–217.

MacKenzie, R.A. (1973, December 3). How to make the most of your time. *U.S. News and World Report,* pp. 45–48, 53–54.

Patrick, P.K.S. (1979). Burnout: Job hazard for health workers. *Hospitals, 53*(22), 87–88, 90.

Predd, C.S. (1982). Setting priorities: How to stay efficient in hectic nursing stations. *Nursing Life, 2*(3), 50–51.

Sa'di [*Gulistan*]. (1970). In R.T. Tripp (Ed.), *The international thesaurus of quotations* (James Ross, Trans.). New York: Crowell. (Original quotation 1258.)

Sanders, M.M. (1980). Stressed or burned out? *The Canadian Nurse, 76*(10), 30–33.

Selye, H. (1976). *Stress in health and disease.* London, Butterworth.

Storlie, F. (1979). Burnout: The elaboration of a concept. *American Journal of Nursing, 79*(2), 2108–2111.

Criteria for Selection of Preceptor

CONSISTENTLY:

1 Assess each patient or admission, using direct and indirect sources of information.
2. Develop a plan of care to assist patient to reach his optimum level of wellness.
3. Implement the plan of care by:
   a. Demonstrating a knowledge of basic nursing skills.
   b. Sustaining and supporting the patient during diagnosis, treatment and rehabilitation.
   c. Facilitating the coordination of health team members.
   d. Identifying learning needs of patients and following through with necessary teaching.
   e. Initiating discharge planning at time of admission.
   f. Demonstrating effective use of hospital and community resources.
   g. Evaluating patient, family response to nursing interventions and making modifications or adaptations in plan of care as a result of the evaluation.
4. Use intellectual, interpersonal and technical skills.
5. Demonstrate ability to identify learning needs of new employees and work with the new employees in devising a plan to meet these needs.
6. Express interest in preceptor role and preceptor program.

From "Preceptors—A Resource for New Nurses" by N. Plasse & J. Lederer, *Supervisor Nurse*, *12*(6), 35. Reprinted by permission.

Orientation Responsibilities Guidelines

	Head Nurse	Preceptor	Nurse Educator	New Employee
Assessment	1. Interviews and hires new employees with input from AHN 2. Administers Clinical Unit Skills Inventory 3. Pre-tests for theory and clinical abilities 4. Compares new employee to competencies in CORE Curriculum	1. Reviews results of and explains use of: • Clinical Skills Inventory • CORE Curriculum • Other tests given with new employees 2. Direct observation of new employee clinical performance	1. Reviews results of: • Clinical Skills Inventory • CORE Curriculum • Other tests given 2. Direct observation of new employee performance	1. Completes and updates Clinical Skills Inventory self assessment of current performance level 2. Identifies own learning needs
Planning	1. Selects preceptor for new employee 2. Informs nursing education, preceptor & unit staff of new employee's hire date and learning needs 3. Assigns new employee to orient day shift and/or off shift	1. Has planning conference with new employee first clinical day 2. Writes mutually agreed upon goals and objectives to increase skill and performance level of new employee	1. Informs preceptor & unit of first clinical day 2. Assists preceptor in writing goals & objectives	1. Writes mutually agreed upon goals and objectives with preceptor
Implementation	1. Provides orientation and preceptor time for new employee	1. Is not "in charge" while precepting 2. Provides learning-center time for new employee 3. Provides learning activities for new employees	1. Provides new employee with general hospital orientation 2. Provides preceptors with preceptor training program 3. Assists preceptor in	1. Reads procedure and policy manuals 2. Initiates own learning experiences 3. Follows learning activities outlined in COPE Curriculum and follows

	4. Acts as clinical resource for new employee 5. Weekly conferences to review progress on technical and process skills 6. Gives ongoing feedback regarding performance 7. Validates skills according to protocol	locating appropriate learning activities	"Guidelines for Integrating Nursing Process into Practice"

Evaluation
 	
1. Evaluates orientee's progress by observation & feedback from orientee & preceptor
2. Conducts 3-month evaluation conference with preceptor and new employee
3. Determines if orientation needs to be extended
4. Assigns new employee to permanent status
	1. Conferences with new employees about progress at end of orientation
	2. Gives feedback to RN regarding new employee's performance
	3. Provides written evaluation to new employee using:
	  — goals & objectives
	  — direct observation
	  — clinical unit skills inventory
	  — Process-to-Practice tool
		1. Assists preceptor & new employee in evaluating new employee's progress
		2. Consults on any proposed extension of probation or orientation
		3. Evaluates orientation and updates learning programs as needed
		4. Reviews orientation evaluation & gives feedback to preceptors and head nurses
			1. Conferences with head nurse and preceptor at end of orientation
			2. Evaluates preceptor program and orientation
			3. Writes self evaluation of progress with use of Clinical Unit Skills Inventory, and mutually set goals & objectives

From *Nursing Decentralization: The El Camino Experience* by Althaus et al., 1981, Rockville, MD: Aspen Systems. Copyright © 1981. Reprinted by permission.

Graduate Nurse Residence Program Plan IV

PROVIDENCE HOSPITAL
Everett, Washington

RESIDENCY PROGRAM

PURPOSE:

To provide an extended clinical experience for the graduate nurse to prepare her for assuming the role of a Registered Nurse in an acute health care facility.

APPLICANTS:

Applicants will be selected from an accredited school of nursing by the Associate Director of Medical-Surgical Nursing on the basis of personal achievement in nursing school and professional attitude toward nursing. Applicants must be able to actively identify their learning needs and be able to prepare independently for the kinds of patients they will be caring for during each segment of the residency. References given by the applicant may be contacted during the interview process. The resident nurse will assume the working schedule of the nursing preceptor(s) to whom she is assigned during the residency period. Ongoing evaluation will occur during the program by the nursing preceptor in cooperation with the Nursing Education Department. The hospital reserves the right to terminate residents who are not meeting the program objectives. A resident who fails to receive a permanent nursing license will also be dropped

Source: Mary Jo Selg, Associate Director, Nursing Education; and Kathryn Morrow, Clinical Educator. Reprinted by permission.

from the program. Applicants must be able to work all shifts during the residency and until a permanent position is found.

Resident will be hired at "graduate nurse-non-licensed" pay scale. Upon receiving license, she will advance to "resident nurse" pay scale. At the end of 11 weeks, resident nurses who have met program objectives will advance to base pay scale and be eligible for benefits as follows: Medical, life and dental insurance and holiday pay. They shall begin accruing sick time and vacation from the date of hire in the Resident Program. The employee may apply or be assigned for open positions in Nursing for the 3 months following the completion of the program. When accepted for a position, this will be considered as a permanent assignment, rather than a transfer. The hospital will also provide references to other facilities at the resident's request.

PROGRAM LENGTH:

11 Weeks

PRECEPTOR SELECTION:

Nursing preceptors will be selected on the recommendation of the unit Head Nurse and willingness of the individual RN to assume this role. The preceptor must be a skilled nurse who demonstrates the nursing process in her practice. It is preferred that the preceptor be a full time staff nurse.

Evaluation Plan: Evaluation will be ongoing by the Resident's preceptor. Preceptors should schedule a weekly (minimum) time to review progress and discuss concerns with the Resident nurse. The Resident will receive a formal evaluation by her preceptor using program objectives at 3, 5, 7, 9, and 11 weeks.

Nursing Education will meet with the residents on a weekly basis to discuss their experiences in the program.

OBJECTIVES FOR NEW NURSING EMPLOYEES

1. State one way that Nursing Philosophy of Providence Hospital will impact nursing care.
2. Describe to whom the nurse is legally accountable for safe nursing practice in the state of Washington.
3. Describe lines of communication for problem-solving within the Nursing organization.
4. State the impact of Providence Hospital Standards of Practice on nursing practice.
5. Define Delivery of Care Systems used at Providence Hospital.
6. Discuss the above concepts in making out an assignment for a sample of patients on Day Shift.

7. Within first three months of employment, complete to the satisfaction of the Head Nurse a Skills Inventory Checklist.
8. State the ways to record continuing education and inservice attendance.
9. Describe how to obtain information on inservice and continuing education opportunities.
10. Define the role of the Infection Control Nurse.
11. Define the procedure for placing a patient on isolation; reporting infection.
12. Recognize containers and know how to collect the following specimens on the unit:
    UA for urinalysis/culture
    Stool
    Sputum for AFB/culture
    Wound culture
13. Locate directions for the various kinds of isolation carried out in the hospital.
14. State the number for Code 4.
15. Describe the location of the Crash Cart for your own unit.
16. Demonstrate the procedure for checking the supplies and equipment on the Crash Cart (return demo on unit) (RN's only).
17. Successfully demonstrate effective CPR.
18. Transcribe correctly a page of MD orders to nursing kardex.
19. Analyze an Admission Assessment (RN's only).
20. Using a sample Admission Assessment, identify patient problems, initiate care plan and SOAP to one problem (RN's only).
21. Demonstrate proper Body Mechanics doing common patient activities.
22. List three services available from Social Services.
23. Review patient policies or procedures on admission, discharge, death, restraints, and bed rails.
24. Demonstrate the steps for safely administering a medication to a patient using the unit dose medication system. (Return demo on unit) (RN's only)
25. State three services provided to patients by the IV Therapy Department.
26. Demonstrate selected functions on the computer system, such as:
    a. Obtaining a patient census.
    b. Obtaining a patient item from CS.
    c. Ordering a patient diet.
    d. Ordering a common laboratory test.

PROGRAM SCHEDULE

WEEK 1:

Hospital and nursing Orientation. Introduction to nursing preceptors. Objectives: See objectives for new nursing employee.

GOALS:

The goal of Weeks 2 and 3 is development of the resident's problem-solving approach to patient care.

WEEK 2:

Resident takes a caseload of 4–5 routine patients under the direction and supervision of the preceptor. Nursing care of these patients should include ongoing assessment; problem identification; goal-setting and planning of care with the patient and his family; carrying out the plan of care including passing their patient's medications; updating care plan and problem-oriented charting. Resident should complete unit scavenger hunt. Completes orientation modules. Completes at least two RN Admission Assessments on routine patients.

WEEK 3:

Takes a caseload of increasingly complex patients applying the nursing process as in Week 2 and continuing to practice new skills as identified by resident on "RN Skills List." Resident should complete RN's Medication Evaluation. Spends one day with Unit Secretary to observe role and complete Computer Skills List. Completes at least two RN Admission Assessments on complex patients.

GOALS:

The goal of Weeks 4 and 5 is for the resident to demonstrate a leadership role in modular nursing and to problem-solve on a larger group of patients.

WEEK 4:

Follows RN Preceptor as she functions in module. Analyzes patient report, leadership and style; learns skills of LPNs or N.A. Assists preceptor with nursing care procedures, documentation and transcription of MD orders. Spends one day observing Head Nurse role.

WEEK 5:

Takes a group of approximately 8 patients under the guidance of her preceptor. Assists Head Nurse or Preceptor in making assignment; receives and gives report; gives care to own patients; makes rounds to assess patients of LPN or NA; identifies priority problems; works with others to implement care; and supervises and directs care given by others. During this time, the resident becomes increasingly independent in function. The preceptor may assume role of consultant, making herself available to residents for questions and discussion while assuming other duties.

GOALS:

The goal of Weeks 6 and 7 is for the resident to demonstrate the RN role on different shifts and to practice problem-solving on a clinically different group of patients.

WEEK 6 & WEEK 7:

Resident rotates to different shift and clinical area. Follows selected LPN for one day to learn shift routine and shift preceptor for 1–2 days to learn leadership routine on that shift and skills of module member(s). Analyzes report and leadership style; assists module members and preceptor in nursing care and documentation.

Takes a module of approximately 8 patients under the guidance of RN preceptor. Receives report; makes rounds to assess patients; identifies priorities; works with staff to implement care; supervises and directs team member(s).

WEEK 8 & WEEK 9:

Resident rotates to different shifts and clinical area. Follows shift preceptor for 1–2 days to learn leadership routine on that shift and skills of module members. Analyzes report and leadership style; assists module and preceptor in nursing care and documentation.

Takes a module under the guidance of RN Preceptor. Receives report; gives care; makes rounds to assess patients, identifies priorities, works with others to implement care, supervises and directs care given by others. Attends codes or traumas as they occur.

WEEK 10 & WEEK 11:

Rotates to different clinical areas. Follows preceptor for 1–2 days to learn routine of floor and skills of module member(s). Assumes leadership role and is expected to function with minimal guidance from preceptor. Resident should utilize this experience to complete remaining skills on RN Skills List.

OPTION:

Residency may be extended to 13 weeks, if appropriate.

FIRST WEEK:

See New Nursing Employee Objectives

2ND WEEK:

1. Shares orientation self-evaluation and RN Skills List with preceptor and identifies nursing skills with which additional experience is needed (assignment should include patients that allow practice of these skills).
2. Demonstrates knowledge of own patients' medications.
3. Demonstrates the correct procedure for administering medications via unit dose delivery system.
4. Demonstrates the correct procedure for administering IV solutions and medications.
5. Updates problem list and care plan of patients to whom assigned.
6. Narrative documentation demonstrates knowledge of SOAP charting format and thoughtful data collection, assessment, and nursing care planning.
7. Identifies patient priorities effectively and organizes work to meet these priorities.
8. Explains logical rationale for priority-setting to preceptor when requested.
9. Demonstrates interview techniques directed toward development of therapeutic relationships with patients to whom assigned.
10. Assists preceptor and other staff willingly.
11. Explains rationale and expected results of nursing and medical treatments in patients being cared for.
12. Evaluates and changes nursing plan as necessary.
13. Completes at least two RN Admission Assessments on routine patients, documenting a review of patient's body systems, usual activities of daily living, emotional instructional and social-discharge planning status.

WEEK THREE:

1. Continues to work on objectives 1–13 with a caseload of patients with multiple needs.
2. Completes to satisfaction of preceptor additional skills from RN Skills List.
3. Completes correctly all steps on RN Medication Evaluation for two days.
4. Completes Computer Skills List.
5. Identifies 3 components of Unit Secretary's role.
6. Completes at least two RN Assessments on complex patients, documenting a review of patient body systems, usual activities of daily living, emotional instructional and social-discharge planning status.
7. Initiates a patient problem list directed toward nursing concerns and a care plan on patients she admits.
8. Observes and discusses role of unit secretary in relation to staff RN role.
9. Correctly requisitions patient services via data collection computer system.

WEEK FOUR:

1. Identifies with preceptor information that should be included on shift-to-shift report.
2. Observes leadership routine and discusses these activities with preceptor.
3. Observes report and discusses content and rationale for assignment of workload with preceptor.
4. Assists preceptor in assessment, implementation of care, transcription of MD orders and documentation of care on patients on team.
5. Continues to demonstrate nursing skills to the satisfaction of preceptor.
6. Transcribes physician orders and correctly requisitions patient services.
7. Observes and discusses role of Head Nurse in relation to staff RN role.

WEEK FIVE:

1. Discusses rationale for patient assignment, considering patient need and staff skill level; utilizes LPN/NA skills to highest level possible.
2. Receives and gives a thorough shift-to-shift report utilizing guidelines for shift report.
3. Receives report from LPN or NA throughout and at end of shift as necessary to obtain information about patients.
4. Assists LPN or NA to assess patient throughout shift; observes patient condition and response to plan of care.
5. Sets priorities re: patient needs and carries out nursing actions accordingly including notification of physician when indicated.
6. Delivers medications and IV Therapy to own and LPN or NA patients according to medication and IV Therapy procedures.
7. Assures that care plans and problem lists on patients are accurate and up-to-date.
8. Charts accurately on those patients for which she is responsible for documentation utilizing SOAP format; co-signs charts for LPNs after checking for completeness and accuracy.
9. Initiates or assures that patient or family instructional needs are assessed and teaching implemented and documented as necessary.
10. Assesses patient's social-discharge planning status early and initiates discharge planning early in patient's stay when appropriate.
11. Initiates discussions with LPN/NA as appropriate to improve skills or change behavior.
12. Completes a transfer summary for a patient being transferred to a nursing home or extended care facility.
13. Adjusts patient care assignments/tasks throughout day to adapt to changes in patient numbers and conditions.
14. Seeks out and provides feedback to preceptor.

15. Demonstrates increasing independence in decision-making and planning, implementation, and evaluation of nursing care.

WEEKS 6 & 7, 8 & 9; and 10 & 11:

1. Repeats objectives for Weeks 4, 5, and 6 with emphasis on new shift and/or different clinical caseload.
2. Completes to satisfaction of preceptor additional skills from RN Skills List.

RESIDENT _____
PRECEPTOR _____
DATE _____
WEEKS 2 and 3
EVALUATION FORM

	Performed Consistently	Often Performed	Occasionally	Seldom or Never Performed	COMMENTS (Use e.g. or expand as needed)
1. Identifies nursing skills with which additional experience is needed. (Preceptor should initial appropriate column(s) on skills list.)					
2. Demonstrates knowledge of own patients' medications.					
3. Demonstrates the correct procedure for administering medications via unit dose delivery system.					
4. Demonstrates the correct procedure for administering IV solutions and medications.					
5. Updates problem list and care plan of patients to whom assigned.					
6. Narrative documentation demonstrates knowledge of SOAP charting format and thoughtful data collection, assessments, and nursing care planning.					
7. Identifies patient priorities effectively and organizes work to meet these priorities.					
8. Explains logical rationale for priority-setting to preceptor when requested.					
9. Demonstrates interview techniques directed toward development of therapeutic relationships with patients to whom she is assigned.					
10. Assists preceptor and other staff members willingly.					
11. Can explain rationale and expected results of nursing and medical treatments in patients being cared for.					
12. Evaluates and changes nursing plan as necessary.					
13. Initiates a patient problem list directed toward nursing concerns and a care plan on patients she admits.					

	Performed Consistently	Often Performed	Occasionally	Seldom or Never Performed	COMMENTS (Use e.g. or expand as needed)
RESIDENT _____ PRECEPTOR _____ DATE _____ WEEKS 2 and 3 EVALUATION FORM					
14. Completes Computer Skills List.					
15. Identifies at least 3 components of Unit Secretary's role.					
16. Completes at least 4 Admission Assessments—two on routine patients, two on complex patients.					

SPECIFIC GOALS:

WEEKS 2 & 3: _____
_____
_____

WEEKS 4 & 5: _____
_____
_____

WEEK _____
_____
_____
_____

STRENGTHS: _____
_____
_____
_____

AREAS NEEDED TO IMPROVE: _____
_____
_____
_____

Signature of Preceptor _____

RESIDENT COMMENTS: _____
_____
_____

Signature of Resident _____

	Performed Consistently	Often Performed	Occasionally	Seldom or Never Performed	COMMENTS (Use e.g. or expand as needed)
RESIDENT _____ PRECEPTOR _____ DATE _____ WEEKS: __ 4 & 5 __ 6 & 7 __ 8 & 9 __ 10 & 11 EVALUATION					
1. Identified with preceptor information that should be included on shift-to-shift report.					
2. Observed routine activities and discussed these with preceptor.					
3. Transcribed physician orders and correctly requisitioned patient services.					
4. Observed and discussed role of Head Nurse in relation to staff nurse role.					
5. Received and gave a thorough shift-to-shift report utilizing guidelines for shift report.					
6. Discussed rationale for patient assignment for module and unit, considered patient need and staff skill level.					
7. Discussed plan for day and assignment with LPN or NA.					
8. Received report from LPN or NA throughout and at end of shift as necessary to obtain information about patients.					
9. Assisted LPN or NA to assess patient throughout shift; observed patient conditions and responses to plan of care.					
10. Set priorities re: patient needs and carried out nursing actions accordingly including notification of physician when indicated.					
11. Delivered medications and IV Therapy to own and LPN/NA's patients according to medication and IV Therapy procedures.					
12. Assured that care plans and problem lists on patients were accurate and up-to-date.					

RESIDENT _____

PRECEPTOR _____

DATE _____

WEEKS: ___ 4 & 5   ___ 6 & 7   ___ 8 & 9
        ___ 10 & 11

EVALUATION

	Performed Consistently	Often Performed	Occasionally	Seldom or Never Performed	COMMENTS (Use e.g. or expand as needed)
13. Charted accurately on those patients for which responsible for documentation utilizing SOAP format.					
14. Cosigned charts of LPNs after checking for completeness and accuracy.					
15. Initiated or assured that patient or family instructional needs were assessed and teaching implemented and documented as necessary.					
16. Assessed patient's social-discharge planning status early and initiated discharge planning early in patient's stay when appropriate.					
17. Completed a transfer summary for patient being transferred to extended care or nursing home (once only).					
18. Initiated discussions with LPNs/NAs as appropriate to improve skills or change behavior.					
19. Completed to satisfaction of preceptor additional skills from RN Skills List (preceptor should initial those skills discussed or demonstrated and those performed).					
20. Adjusted patient care assignments/tasks throughout day to adapt to changes in patient numbers and conditions.					

STRENGTHS: _____

_____

_____

AREAS NEEDED TO IMPROVE: _____

_____

_____

_____

                        Signature of Preceptor _____

RESIDENT COMMENTS: _____

_____

_____

_____

_____

                        Signature of Resident _____

Instrumentation of the Taxonomy of Educational Objectives

Cognitive Domain

Taxonomy	Classification	Examples of Infinitives	KEY WORDS Examples of Direct Objects
1.00	Knowledge		
1.10	Knowledge of Specifics		
1.11	Knowledge of Terminology	to define, to distinguish, to acquire, to identify, to recall, to recognize	vocabulary, terms, terminology, meaning(s), definitions, referents, elements
1.12	Knowledge of Specific Facts	to recall, to recognize, to acquire, to identify	facts, factual information, (sources), (names), (dates), (events), (persons), (places), (time periods), properties, examples, phenomena
1.20	Knowledge of Ways and Means of Dealing with Specifics		
1.21	Knowledge of Conventions	to recall, to identify, to recognize, to acquire	forms, convention(s), uses, usage, rules, ways, devices, symbols, representations, style(s), formats

From *Perspectives in Individualized Learning* (pp. 189–192) by R.A. Weisgerber, 1971, Itasca, IL: Peacock. Copyright © 1971. Reprinted by permission.

Taxonomy	Classification	*KEY WORDS* Examples of Infinitives	Examples of Direct Objects
1.22	Knowledge of Trends, Sequences	to recall, to recognize, to acquire, to identify	action(s), processes, movement(s), continuity, development(s), trend(s), sequence(s), causes, relationship(s), forces, influences
1.23	Knowledge of Classifications and Categories	to recall, to recognize, to acquire, to identify	area(s), type(s), feature(s), class(es), set(s), division(s), arrangement(s), classification(s), category/categories
1.24	Knowledge of Criteria	to recall, to recognize, to acquire, to identify,	criteria, basics, elements
1.25	Knowledge of Methodology	to recall, to recognize, to acquire, to identify	methods, techniques, approaches, uses, procedures, treatments
1.30	Knowledge of the Universals and Abstractions in a Field		
1.31	Knowledge of Principles, Generalizations	to recall, to recognize, to acquire, to identify	principle(s), generalization(s), proposition(s), fundamentals, laws, principal elements, implications
1.32	Knowledge of Theories and Structures	to recall, to recognize, to acquire, to identify	theories, bases, interrelations, structure(s), organization(s), formulation(s)
2.00	Comprehension		
2.10	Translation	to translate, to transform, to give in own words, to illustrate, to prepare, to read, to represent, to change, to rephrase, to restate	meaning(s), sample(s), definitions, abstractions, representations, words, phrases

		KEY WORDS	
Taxonomy	Classification	*Examples of Infinitives*	*Examples of Direct Objects*

Taxonomy	Classification	Examples of Infinitives	Examples of Direct Objects
2.20	Interpretation	to interpret, to reorder, to rearrange, to differentiate, to distinguish, to make, to draw, to explain, to demonstrate	relevancies, relationships, essentials, aspects, new view(s), qualifications, conclusions, methods, theories, abstractions
2.30	Extrapolation	to estimate, to infer, to conclude, to predict, to differentiate, to determine, to extend, to interpolate, to extrapolate, to fill in, to draw	consequences, implications, conclusions, factors, ramifications, meanings, corollaries, effects, probabilities
3.00	Application	to apply, to generalize, to relate, to choose, to develop, to organize, to use, to employ, to transfer, to restructure, to classify	principles, laws, conclusions, effects, methods, theories, abstractions, situations, generalizations, processes, phenomena, procedures
4.00	Analysis		
4.10	Analysis of Elements	to distinguish, to detect, to identify, to classify, to discriminate, to recognize, to categorize, to deduce	elements, hypothesis/hypotheses, conclusions, assumptions, statements (of fact), statements (of intent), arguments, particulars
4.20	Analysis of Relationships	to analyze, to contrast, to compare, to distinguish, to deduce	relationships, interrelations, relevance, relevancies, themes, evidence, fallacies, arguments, cause-effect(s), consistency/consistencies, parts, ideas, assumptions
4.30	Analysis of Organizational Principles	to analyze, to distinguish, to detect, to deduce	form(s), pattern(s), purpose(s), point(s) of view(s), techniques, bias(es), structure(s), theme(s), arrangement(s), organization(s)

Taxonomy	Classification	KEY WORDS Examples of Infinitives	Examples of Direct Objects
5.0	Synthesis		
5.10	Production of a Unique Communication	to write, to tell, to relate, to produce, to constitute, to transmit, to originate, to modify, to document	structure(s), pattern(s), product(s), performance(s), design(s), work(s), communications, effort(s), specifics, composition(s)
5.20	Production of a Plan, or Proposed Set of Operations	to propose, to plan, to produce, to design, to modify, to specify	plan(s), objectives, specification(s), schematic(s), operations, way(s), solution(s), means
5.30	Derivation of a Set of Abstract Relations	to produce, to derive, to develop, to combine, to organize, to synthesize, to classify, to deduce, to formulate, to modify	phenomena, taxonomies, concept(s), scheme(s), theories, relationships, abstractions, generalizations, hypothesis/hypotheses, perceptions, ways, discoveries
6.00	Evaluation		
6.10	Judgments in Terms of Internal Evidence	to judge, to argue, to validate, to assess, to decide	accuracy/accuracies, consistency/consistencies, fallacies, reliability, flaws, errors, precision, exactness
6.20	Judgments in Terms of External Criteria	to judge, to argue, to consider, to compare, to contrast, to standardize, to appraise	ends, means, efficiency, economy/economies, utility, alternatives, courses of action, standards, theories, generalizations

Affective Domain

Taxonomy	Classification	Examples of Infinitives	Examples of Direct Objects
1.0	Receiving		
1.1	Awareness	to differentiate, to separate, to set apart, to share	sights, sounds, events, designs, arrangements
1.2	Willingness to Receive	to accumulate, to select, to combine, to accept	models, examples, shapes, sizes, meters, cadences
1.3	Controlled or Selected Attention	to select, to posturally respond to, to listen (for), to control	alternatives, answers, rhythms, nuances
2.0	Responding		
2.1	Acquiescence	to comply (with), to follow, to commend, to approve	directions, instructions, laws, policies, demonstrations
2.2	Willingness to Respond	to volunteer, to discuss, to practice, to play	instruments, games, dramatic works, charades, burlesques
2.3	Satisfaction in Response	to applaud, to acclaim, to spend leisure time in, to augment	speeches, plays, presentations, writings
3.0	Valuing		
3.1	Acceptance of a Value	to increase measured proficiency in, to increase numbers of, to relinquish, to specify	group membership(s), artistic production(s), musical productions, personal friendships
3.2	Preference for a Value	to assist, to subsidize, to help, to support	artists, projects, viewpoints, arguments
3.3	Commitment	to deny, to protest, to debate, to argue	deceptions, irrelevancies, abdications, irrationalities
4.0	Organization		

Taxonomy	Classification	Examples of Infinitives	Examples of Direct Objects
4.1	Conceptualization of a Value	to discuss, to theorize (on), to abstract, to compare	parameters, codes, standards goals
4.2	Organization of a Value System	to balance, to organize, to define, to formulate	systems, approaches, criteria, limits
5.0	Characterization by Value or Value Complex		
5.1	Generalized Set	to revise, to change, to complete, to require	plans, behavior, methods, efforts
5.2	Characterization	to be rated high by peers in, to be rated high by superiors in, to be rated high by subordinates in	humanitarianism, ethics, integrity, maturity
		and	
		to avoid, to manage, to resolve, to resist	extravagance(s), excesses, conflicts, exorbitancy/ exorbitancies

Novice Position Description

PROVIDENCE HOSPITAL   POSITION DESCRIPTION
Everett, Washington

Department: NURSING SERVICE   Date:
Position Title: RESIDENT REGISTERED NURSE
Position Number:

SUMMARY

A registered nurse or new graduate nurse whose clinical experience after graduation is less than 12 months; or a Registered Nurse who is returning to practice with no current clinical training and experience. He/she is responsible for an assigned group of patients who require skilled care and observation. He/she cares for these patients under close supervision of an experienced R.N. preceptor.

POSITION FUNCTIONS

IS ABLE TO INTERPRET NURSING POLICIES AND SUPPORT OR-GANIZATIONAL STRUCTURE WHICH DELINEATES FUNCTIONS AND CHANNELS OF COMMUNICATION WITHIN NURSING SERVICE.

Accepts and utilizes the philosophy and nursing objectives of Nursing Service and his/her unit in his/her relationship with personnel, patients and family.

Source: Providence Hospital, Everett, Washington. Reprinted by permission.

Fosters cooperative effort through understanding the functions of all personnel involved in patient care.

Participates in the review and revision of position description for the Resident Registered Nurse and Registered Nurse.

Interprets and utilizes the organizational chart showing channels of communication within Nursing Service.

Keeps charge or Head Nurse informed of progress in performance of functions.

Functions within established or revised nursing personnel policies.

After a designated period of orientation, instruction and competence demonstration, is able to assume the duties of modular, total patient care or primary nursing, assuming a caseload of patients under the supervision of another experienced Registered Nurse, which may be the Supervisor or Head Nurse.

GIVES SAFE AND EFFECTIVE NURSING CARE.

Responsible for seeing that treatments are administered.

Provides physical and emotional comfort and safety for his/her patients.

Takes initiative in participating and sharing information in the establishment, implementation and evaluation of nursing care plans.

Consults with the experienced Registered Nurse, Supervisor or Head Nurse when in doubt or in need of help.

Leads or participates in patient conferences.

Determines personal competence in performing nursing functions and seeks guidance when necessary.

Sets an example of professional skill and performance to other members of the nursing staff.

Responsible that the needs of each newly admitted or fresh post-operative patient assigned to him/her are assessed and recorded on the nursing care plan.

Responsible for the physical and mental preparation of his/her assigned patients for surgery, tests or procedures.

Responsible for maintenance of parenteral fluids on his/her assigned patients.

Sets an example to other staff members by properly utilizing techniques, procedures and equipment.

Participates in patient and family teaching.

Makes suggestions for improving patient care.

KEEPS COMPLETE, ACCURATE AND CONCISE CLINICAL NURSING RECORDS AND REPORTS.

Is responsible for own clinical recording and reporting.

Observes procedures and policies pertaining to any aspect of clinical charting and reporting.

Suggests methods of improving charting and reporting.

Responsible that nursing care plans of patients under their care are updated and available for use by other members of the nursing staff.

Responsible for keeping the preceptor, charge nurse or Head Nurse informed of the condition of his/her patients.

ASSISTS IN PLANNING AND DECISION-MAKING WHICH EFFECTS THE OPERATION OF THE NURSING DEPARTMENT AND THE CARE OF PATIENTS.

Applies policies governing the use of hospital facilities, patients and nursing personnel by schools of nursing.

Assists unit staff and Head Nurse in planning for adequate facilities, equipment and supplies which influence the performance of nursing personnel.

Cooperates with other departments in providing care for patients assigned.

Participates in designated committees directed toward the fulfillment of the Nursing Service objectives.

FUNCTIONS WITHIN A BUDGET WHICH IS SUFFICIENT FOR THE PROVISION OF QUALITY NURSING CARE.

Is able to interpret the budget to other nursing staff and encourages economical use of supplies and equipment.

Organizes work schedule to make optimum use of his/her time and ability.

Works and plans with other nursing staff for time when cooperative effort is needed.

PROMOTES AND PARTICIPATES IN EDUCATIONAL NURSING OP-PORTUNITIES FOR THE DEVELOPMENT OF SELF AND OTHER NURS-ING PERSONNEL.

Suggests and participates in inservice educational programs geared to meet the needs of self.

Is able to evaluate with aide of preceptor, Head Nurse, Supervisor and others what type of further education he/she needs and seeks to obtain this education.

Keeps abreast and shares knowledge of current nursing trends and developments gained by reading and participating in educational opportunities outside the hospital.

Seeks learning opportunities and shares pertinent information with others.

Fosters creativity and recommends ideas which benefit Nursing Service and the patient.

Assists unit staff and Head Nurse in orientation of new personnel when possible.

PARTICIPATES IN SELF EVALUATION OF NURSING PERFORMANCE AND IN MAINTAINING RECORDS PERTINENT TO SELF.

Confers at designated intervals with preceptor and Head Nurse for written self-evaluation and conference.

Utilizes evaluation for maintaining or improving personal performance and ability to take on greater responsibility.

Notifies appropriate person of changes in personal status.

Responsible that incident reports involving self are accurate and complete.

CONTINUALLY EVALUATES THE EFFECT OF NURSING SERVICE GIVEN TO PATIENT BY SELF AND NURSING PERSONNEL.

Participates in review and/or revision of existing policies and functions of nursing as designated by the Head Nurse.

Supports changes which benefit Nursing Service.

Participates in individual and group conferences for approval of functions and personnel inter-relationships of the nursing staff.

PERFORMS ASSOCIATED FUNCTIONS AS REQUESTED.

QUALIFICATIONS

Graduate of an accredited school of nursing.

Currently (or temporarily as in the case of the new graduate) licensed to practice as a Registered Nurse in the State of Washington.

Professional attributes as stated in the "Code for Professional Nurses."

Ability to adapt emotional responses to the needs of the situation.

Willingness to learn and use every opportunity to improve his/her nursing skills.

Knowledge and ability to apply the correct nursing techniques and practices for which he/she has been prepared.

Ability to actively identify his/her learning needs and be able to prepare independently for the kinds of patients they will be caring for during each segment of the residency.

POSITION RELATIONSHIPS

Supervised by: The assigned preceptor and the Head Nurse.

Persons supervised: None.

Guide for Planning Settings

Purpose of Offering	Method	Setting
Information giving	Lecture	Auditorium
	Panel	Classroom
	Institute	Auditorium
	Self-instruction	Carrel
Problem-solving	Seminar	Conference
	Conference	Rounds
	Case study	Squares
	Learning games	Conference
	Self-instruction	Carrel
Skill development (procedures equipment, directing others)	Lecture with demonstration	Small auditorium
	Return demonstration	
		Classroom
	Learning games	Conference
	Self-instruction	Carrel

From *The Process of Staff Development: Components for Change* (2nd ed.) (p.150) by H. Tobin, P. Yoder Wise, and P. Hull, 1979, St. Louis: Mosby. Copyright © 1979. Reprinted by permission.

Appendix G

Evaluation Forms for Preceptor Program Graduate Nurse Residency

EVALUATION OF PROGRAM
GRADUATE NURSE RESIDENCY

1. Do you feel you learned from this program?

___ Nothing   Comments _____
___ Review of material   _____
___ Learned some new material   _____
___ Learned much new material   _____

2. Did the program cover the content you expected?

___ Yes   Comments _____
___ No   _____
    _____
    _____

3. Do you feel you have increased/improved your technical skills?

___ Not at all   Comments _____
___ Some   _____
___ A great deal   _____

4. Do you feel you have increased/improved your use of nursing process?

___ Not at all   Comments _____
___ Some   _____
___ A great deal   _____

Source: Providence Hospital, Everett, Washington. Reprinted by permission.

5. Do you feel you have increased/improved your interpersonal/communication skills?

    _____ Not at all   Comments _____
    _____ Some   _____
    _____ A great deal   _____

6. Were the teaching methods and materials effective for your learning?

    _____ Yes   _____ No

7. If not, what methods or materials would have increased your learning?

    _____
    _____

8. Did your preceptors provide professional models for your practice?

    _____ Yes   Comments _____
    _____ No   _____
                                       _____

9. Did the meetings with Nursing Education meet your needs? Do you have suggestions for improvement?

    _____
    _____
    _____

10. How was the length of the program?

    _____ Too long
    _____ Too short
    _____ About right

11. Has the residency facilitated your transition from student to professional nurse? How?

12. Has the residency program met your expectations overall, and do you feel comfortable in assuming a staff nurse role?

13. Do you have suggestions that might help to improve the program for future groups?

14. Additional Comments:

PRECEPTOR EVALUATION OF PROGRAM
GRADUATE NURSE RESIDENCY

1. Do you feel that, overall, the residency program benefits new graduates?

   _____ Yes   Comments _____

   _____ No   _____

   _____ Only a little _____

2. Does the program cover the content you expect?

   _____ Yes   Comments _____

   _____ No   _____

   _____

3. Do you feel the residents increase/improve their technical skills?

   _____ Not at all   Comments _____

   _____ Some   _____

   _____ A great deal _____

4. Do you feel the residents increase/improve their use of nursing process?

   _____ Not at all   Comments _____

   _____ Some   _____

   _____ A great deal _____

5. Do you feel the residents increase/improve their interpersonal and communication skills?

   _____ Not at all   Comments _____

   _____ Some   _____

   _____ A great deal _____

6. Do you feel the residents increase/improve their teaching skills?

   _____ Not at all   Comments _____

   _____ Some   _____

   _____ A great deal _____

7. If not, what methods or materials would increase their learning?

   _____

8. How is the length of the program?

   _____ Too long

   _____ Too short

   _____ About right

9. Does the residency facilitate transition from student to professional nurse? How?

10. Do you have suggestions that might help to improve the program for future groups?

11. As a preceptor, what information or resources would you find useful in helping your residents or improving your skills as a preceptor?

12. Additional Comments:

MANAGEMENT EVALUATION OF PROGRAM
GRADUATE NURSE RESIDENCY

1. Do you feel that, overall, the residency program benefits new graduates?

    _____ Yes   Comments _____

    _____ No   _____

    _____ Only a little   _____

2. Does the program cover the content you expect?

    _____ Yes   Comments _____

    _____ No   _____

                             _____

3. Do you feel the residents increase/improve their technical skills?

    _____ Not at all   Comments _____

    _____ Some   _____

    _____ A great deal   _____

4. Do you feel the residents increase/improve their use of nursing process?

    _____ Not at all   Comments _____

    _____ Some   _____

    _____ A great deal   _____

5. Do you feel the residents increase/improve their interpersonal and communication skills?

    _____ Not at all   Comments _____

    _____ Some   _____

    _____ A great deal   _____

6. Do you feel the residents increase/improve their teaching skills?

    _____ Not at all   Comments _____

    _____ Some   _____

    _____ A great deal   _____

7. Do you feel the preceptor (buddy) system is effective for 1:1 teaching/ learning? If not, what would work better?

    _____ Yes   Comments _____

    _____ No   _____

                               _____

8. Do you find the residency program weekly objectives appropriate for the residents?

    _____ Yes   Comments _____   _____

    _____ No   _____   _____

                               _____   _____

9. Are you familiar with the evaluation forms?   _____   _____ No

    Are they adequate? If not, how should they be changed?

    _____ Yes   Comments _____   _____

    _____ No   _____   _____

                               _____   _____

10. How is the length of the program?

    _____ Too long

    _____ Too short

    _____ About right

11. Do you feel the residency facilitates transition from student to professional nurse? How?

12. Do you have suggestions that might help to improve the program for future groups?

Case Study Guidelines

CASE STUDY GUIDELINES
Learner

1. What are the physical needs of the patient?
   Consider: Activity/rest; comfort; communications; elimination; growth and development; nutrition; oxygenation; protection/safety; sleep/wake.
2. What are the psycho-social needs of the patient?
   Consider: Self-concept; emotional status; behavior; response to stress (coping and defense mechanisms); interpersonal relationships; life style (occupational and family roles); dependence/independence; economic factors.
3. What is the patient's cognitive-perceptual state?
   Consider: Educational level; intellectual function (thought processes, verbal abilities); language skills; learning needs; expectations of self, nurses and physicians; perceptual difficulties (vision, hearing, etc.)
4. Have cultural-spiritual needs been considered?
   Consider: Religious preference and importance; country of origin; ceremonies or routines important to the patient because of religion or nationality.
5. What are the pertinent needs/nursing diagnoses for this patient?
   Consider: Problem, etiology and presenting signs and symptoms.
6. What are realistic goals for this patient?
   Consider: severity of pathology; likelihood of progression or remission; patient's motivation, capabilities and perceptions; available resources and/ or technology.
7. Have available resources been considered?
   Consider: In-house resources (occupational therapy, physical therapy, respiratory therapy, etc.); outside resources (Reach-to-recover, Alcoholics Anonymous, etc.); patient support systems (family, friends, organizations); patient's own motivation, talents and strengths.

8. What are your learning needs regarding this patient?
Consider: Familiarity with diagnosis and modes of treatment; information from patient, staff and physicians.
9. Have you taken advantage of the opportunities for teaching or communicating with others about this patient?
Consider: Patient; family/significant other; nursing and non-nursing staff; physician; outside resources.

CASE STUDY GUIDELINES
Instructor

1. What are the physical needs of the patient?
What are the physical needs of the patient based on your assessment? Which needs are not being met? What are the potential problems? Does your care plan reflect these? Consider: Activity/rest; comfort; communications; elimination; growth and development; nutrition; oxygenation; protection/safety; sleep/wake.
2. What are the psycho-social needs of the patient?
How does the patient normally spend his day? What is the impact of hospitalization? Is protection from environmental stimulation or excessive numbers of people needed? Is more stimulation needed? What is the patient's independence level? Is a coordinated approach needed from staff to manage manipulative behavior? Are you aware of the patient's emotional state? Are opportunities for verbalization provided? What are the relationships between the patient and family members, staff, physician? What are the patient's usual coping mechanisms? Are they working, or is intervention needed? Is the patient concerned about family at home, finances, or job?
3. What is the patient's cognitive-perceptual state?
What is the patient's understanding of his disease state? What are his/her expectations of self and the health care providers? Are there physical, perceptual or psycho-social factors which influence interactions and understanding? What are the patient's learning needs? Have discharge needs been considered?
4. Have cultural-spiritual needs been considered?
Have cultural or religious factors which are important to the patient or which influence hospitalization been considered and incorporated into the plan of care where possible?
5. What are the pertinent needs/nursing diagnoses for this patient?
Have all of the areas above been considered? What are the priorities for action? Have the diagnoses been validated with the patient?

6. What are realistic goals for this patient?
   What are realistic goals for this patient? Have you discussed these goals with the physician and other health care team members? Have diagnosis, severity, motivation and capabilities been considered? Are you comfortable with these goals or will you feel defeated?

Preceptor Workshop Example

PRINCIPLES FOR PRECEPTORS

COURSE DESCRIPTION

A two day Workshop designed for staff nurses functioning as "Preceptors" with acute or critical care resident nurses here at Providence. The Workshop will assist the experienced R.N. to develop his or her skills as a preceptor.

The Workshop will focus on:

1. The Preceptor Role
2. Communication Skills/Conflict Resolution
3. Role Relationships/Relationship Building
4. Identifying and Managing Stress as a Preceptor or Resident
5. Teaching/Learning Principles of Adult Education
6. Planning/Time Management
7. Teaching Techniques
8. Performance Evaluation
   DATES:
   TIME:
   LOCATION:
   REGISTRATION:
   (Limited to 30 participants)

PROGRAM OBJECTIVES

FIRST DAY:

1. List at least four components of a preceptor's role.
2. Explain role socialization as it relates to self and orientee.

3. Discuss the role relationship between:
    a. preceptor-orientee
    b. preceptor-peers
    c. orientee-peers
    d. head nurse/charge nurse/team leader/orientee/preceptor
    e. orientee—health team member
    as they affect establishment of the orientee's identity.
4. Identify at least four factors which may stress preceptor and/or orientee; recognize behavior cues that would aid in identification of the stressor and select possible strategies for stress reduction.
5. Examine own communication style and methods to enhance communication between self and others.
6. Identify conflict promoting behaviors and demonstrate a specific strategy useful for conflict resolution.

SECOND DAY:

1. Identify criteria for effective teaching.
2. Utilize a clinical teaching self assessment form to identify own areas of strength and need regarding teaching.
3. List at least four principles of adult education; distinguish between adult and children's learning styles.
4. Identify value of program planning as essential step to successful program outcome.
5. Identify at least two strategies for effective time management on clinical unit.
6. Identify and discuss the influence of five verbal and non-verbal behaviors on teacher-student interactions.
7. Identify and discuss at least two strategies suitable for one-to-one teaching.
8. Differentiate between behavior descriptions and judgments about behavior.
9. Establish a systematic approach to recording behavior descriptions for use in performance evaluation.

PRECEPTOR WORKSHOP OUTLINE

Day 1:	I. Program Overview	Lecture	10 minutes
	II. The Preceptor Role	Group discussion with faculty facilitator	45 minutes
	III. Preceptor Skills	Lecture/Discussion—self-assessment tool	30 minutes
	IV. Communication Skills	Lecture/Role play/Small group activities	2 hours, 15 minutes

	V.	Roles & Relationships	Lecture/Discussion/ Small groups	1 hour, 30 minutes
	VI.	Stress Identification	Lecture with group partici- pation	45 minutes
	VII.	Stress Management	Lecture/Demonstration/ Role Plays	1 hour, 15 minutes
Day 2:	I.	Criteria for Effective Teaching/ Learning	Group participation with fac- ulty facilitator	20 minutes
	II.	Clinical Teaching Skills	Written self-assessment tool	20 minutes
	III.	Principles of Adult Edu- cation	Lecture with Audio-visual aids	1 hour
	IV.	Planning Learning Activ- ities	Lecture with tool examples	45 minutes
	V.	Time management	Lecture with Audio-visual aids	45 minutes
	VI.	Teacher Tactics	Lecture/Role play/ Demonstration	2 hours
	VII.	Performance Review Evaluation	Lecture/Practice	1 hour 15 minutes

Exercises for Giving Criticism

TAKING RESPONSIBILITY FOR ONE'S POSITIONS OR FEELINGS

Responsibility Not Taken	*Responsibility Taken*
You should exercise every day.	I have found I feel much better if I get some exercise every day.
Everyone thought your speech was great.	I really feel what you had to say was tremendous.
Our boss doesn't listen to us enough.	I would really like it if our boss would spend some time with me individually.
No one likes to talk about their personal life.	I am not comfortable discussing my personal life.

Now, in your small groups, rewrite the following, changing each from impersonal, generalized statements to ones which express where the speaker is; from "disowned" to "owned" statements. Verbally describe as explicitly as you can the feelings that might be behind each statement.

You are always too busy to listen.

_____

You think only about yourself.

_____

Everyone feels you are too bossy.

_____

_____

Source: Cheryl Kilbourn. Reprinted by permission.

You're wrong about that!

Oh, come on. How can you say THAT?

That was a boring meeting.

It's so nice to have you here working with us.

Why don't you ever say anything?

Someone should tell Martha that she monopolizes the conversation.

BASED ON GUIDELINES, WHAT IS WRONG WITH THESE STATE-MENTS?

1. You don't have the right attitude.

---

2. You should be more careful.

---

3. You're always late.

---

4. You are a bad boy (or girl).

---

5. You should get your homework done early when you get home from school like your sister does.

---

6. You're a real troublemaker and you are insensitive to others. And, you're always late and you always interrupt people.

---

7. You never listen to me.

---

8. Everyone says you are too bossy.

---

9. You're never home in time for dinner.

---

10. You always exaggerate everything.

---

11. You think only about yourself.

---

12. Why did you talk to John that way this morning? (using negative tone)

---

13. Every time I ask you to do something I have to repeat it 3 times.

---

14. Everyone thinks you're undependable.

---

15. You were really stupid yesterday. (person knows what critic is referring to)

Preceptor Assessment Tools

SELF-EVALUATION

I. Am I familiar with the facility?

Yes	No		
___	___	Philosophy	Comments _____
___	___	Goals and objectives	_____
___	___	Organizational structure	_____
___	___	Physical facility	_____
___	___	Committees	_____
___	___	Medical staff	_____
___	___	Other	_____

II. Am I familiar with the department?

___	___	Philosophy	Comments _____
___	___	Goals and objectives	_____
___	___	Organization	_____
___	___	Committees	_____
___	___	Other	_____

III. Am I familiar with the unit?

___	___	Philosophy	Comments _____
___	___	Goals and objectives	_____
___	___	Delivery of care method (primary, team, etc.)	_____
___	___	Floor plan	_____
___	___	Daily routines	_____
___	___	Payroll system	_____
___	___	Operation and trouble-shooting of equipment	_____

_____	_____	Emergency protocols (fire,disaster, codes, etc.)	_____
_____	_____	Inservices and continuing education	_____
_____	_____	Certification programs	_____
_____	_____	Time schedules and requests	_____
_____	_____	Medication system	_____
_____	_____	Communication systems	_____
_____	_____	Admission, discharge, transfer and post mortem procedures	_____
_____	_____	Location of equipment especially emergency equipment	_____

IV. Am I familiar with resources?

_____	_____	Policy/procedure books	Comments _____
_____	_____	Clinical specialists	_____
_____	_____	Staff development department	_____
_____	_____	Manuals from other departments	_____

V. Am I familiar with the novice's program?

_____	_____	My role	Comments _____
_____	_____	Role and responsibility of program coordinator/staff development department	_____
_____	_____	Novice responsibilities	_____
_____	_____	Purpose and objectives	_____
_____	_____	Plan and timetable	_____
_____	_____	Evaluation system	_____
_____	_____	When and how to refer problems or concerns	_____

PRECEPTOR SELF-EVALUATION

Identify each of the following according to your need for information.

I. Teaching

_____ Assessing novice's learning needs
_____ Assisting novice to set realistic personal goals
_____ Using principles of adult learning
_____ Organizing material to be presented or discussed
_____ Assisting novice to build needed skills and knowledge
_____ Using graded approach in teaching (simple to complex, known to unknown)
_____ Emphasizing novice's ability to develop solutions rather than providing them
_____ Remaining calm, composed and non-judgmental
_____ Recognizing effectiveness of instruction and modifying approach as needed
_____ Establishing a climate of mutual respect and trust
_____ Writing evaluations

II. Consulting

_____ Acquainting novice with and/or interpreting policies/procedures and protocols
_____ Assisting novice to define and assume expected role behaviors
_____ Serving as a resource to the novice
_____ Providing positive and negative feedback
_____ Offering support and encouragement

III. Practice

_____ Keeping current in own area of practice
_____ Responding to others as individuals, not as one in a series
_____ Maintaining own enthusiasm
_____ Modeling professional standards, values and skills
_____ Integrating the "real world" with the ideal
_____ Recognizing my limitations

IV. Research

_____ Using reference materials and persons
_____ Seeking out learning experiences to meet novice's needs and goals

1 = high priority
2 = medium priority
3 = low priority
4 = no need

PRECEPTOR
NEEDS ASSESSMENT CHECKLIST

_____ Communication

_____ Dealing with conflict

_____ Teaching others

_____ Performance Evaluation

_____ Giving criticism

_____ Making patient assignments

_____ Writing objectives

_____ Goal-setting

_____ Reality shock

_____ Dealing with the new
        graduate

_____ How to give praise

_____ Assignments

_____ Guiding and developing
        others

_____ Hospital resources

_____ Stress management

_____ Time management

_____ Crisis intervention

_____ Dealing with anger

_____ Planning for instruction

_____ Teaching methods

_____ Delegation of authority to the
        novice

_____ Directing the work of others

_____ Coaching/Counseling

_____ How to give criticism

_____ Understanding individual
        differences

Please take a moment to check the topics you are interested in learning more about during the next year.

Appendix L

A Management Preceptorship

DESCRIPTION OF PRECEPTORSHIP

Description: Initially, a consolidated four-hour weekly, on-unit experience wherein a staff education faculty member is available as preceptor to the new head nurse, providing guidance, support, and problem-solving assistance. Once the role has been negotiated among the head nurse, the nursing service, and the faculty member, the experience will still be on-unit, but most likely will be spread out—that is, plus or minus one hour in each of several activities, such as helping the head nurse structure an evaluation appraisal, a staff meeting, a service leadership meeting, report, or rounds. However, total weekly involvement should not exceed significantly the four hours, given the faculty member's other job requirements and expectations.

Purpose: To provide the new head nurse with structured management guidance and the faculty member with an appropriate channel through which to fulfill the clinical* component of the position.

Objectives: Upon completion of this experience the participants should be better prepared to:

1. Identify by documented methods the continuous management learning needs of (a) the individual preceptee, and (b) the representative unit.
2. State through various inventories the leadership style of the head nurse.
3. Evaluate the above leadership style through various instruments which allow for self, peer, and staff perceptions.

From *"Developing Head Nurses: One Hospital's Solution"* by J. Garity, 1983, *Nurse Educator,* 9(3), 38–42. Reprinted by permission.
*The definition of *clinical* in our context is "managerial knowledge, skills, and practices."

4. Identify, apply, document, and evaluate various problem-solving/resolving methods in relation to ongoing unit problems, issues, and concerns.

Recommendations/Requirements:

- Evaluate the preceptorship through self, peers, and staff perceptions.
- Submit to the respective nursing chairman a report summarizing the effectiveness of the preceptorship and offering opinions, conclusions, and any proposals for the future.
- Meet prn with head nurse, clinical leader, and preceptor.
- Meet prn with head nurse, clinical leader, chairman and preceptor.
- Provide a bibliography of core leadership readings.
- Provide related assignments.
- Participate in established management programs—e.g. Orientation, Group Dynamics, Evaluation, Assertiveness.

Bibliography

Aime, D.B. (1979). Employee evaluations: What's the difference? *Supervisor Nurse, 10*(6), 52–60.

Alspach, J. (1978). A critical care nursing internship program: Gripping versus griping. *Supervisor Nurse, 9*(9), 31–40.

Althous, J.N., Hardyck, N.M., Pierce, P.B., & Rodgers, M.S. (1981). *Nursing decentralization: The El Camino experience.* Wakefield, MA: Nursing Resources.

Anthony, W.P. (1981). *Managing incompetence.* New York: AMACOM.

Araujo, M. (1980). Creative nursing administration sets climate for retention. *Hospitals, 54*(9), 72–76.

Archbold, C.R. (1977). Our nurse interns are a sound investment. *RN, 40*(9) 105, 107, 109–110, 112.

Atwood, A.H. (1979). The mentor in clinical practice. *Nursing Outlook, 27*(11), 714–717.

Atwood, H., et al. (1971). Concept of need: An analysis for adult education. *Adult Leadership, 19*(1), 212. Cited in D.F. Bell. (1978). Assessing educational needs: Advantages and disadvantages of eighteen techniques. *Nurse Educator, 3*(5), 15–21.

Axford, R.W. (1969). *Adult education: The open door.* Scranton, PA: International Textbook.

Bakker, C.B., & Bakker-Rabdau, M.K. (1973). *No Trespassing! Explorations in human territoriality.* San Francisco: Chandler and Sharp.

Bavaro, J.A. (1980). Questioning: The key to learning. *Supervisor Nurse, 11*(6), 26–28.

Bell, D.F. (1978). Assessing educational needs: Advantages and disadvantages of eighteen techniques. *Nurse Educator, 7*(5), 15–21.

Bell, D.F., & Bell, D.L. (1979). Effective evaluations. *Nurse Educator, 4*(6), 6–15.

Bell, D.F., & Bell, D.L. (1983). Harmonizing self directed and teacher directed approaches to learning. *Nurse Educator, 8*(2), 24–30.

Benner, P. (1982). From novice to expert. *American Journal of Nursing, 82*(3), 402–407.

Bevis, E.O. (1978). *Curriculum building in nursing: A process* (2nd ed.). St. Louis: Mosby.

Birdzell, J.R. (1975). The transition from subordinate to supervisor. *Hospital Topics, 53*(6), 20–22.

Blanchard, K., & Johnson, S. (1982). *The one minute manager.* New York: Morrow.

Blanchard, S.L. (1983). The discontinuity between school & practice. *Nursing Management, 14*(4), 41–43.

265

Bloom, S. (1956). *Taxonomy of educational objectives: The classification of educational goals. Handbook I: Cognitive domain.* New York: David McKay.

Bogner, H. (1982). How to keep the nurses you hire. *Nursing Life*, 2(6), 18.

Bomberger, A.S., & Kern, C.J. (1982). MIC: A self-directed learning method for nursing staff. *Nurse Educator*, 7(4), 30–31.

Bower, F.L. (1974). Normative or criterion referenced evaluation? *Nursing Outlook*, 22(8), 499–502.

Bransom, R.M. (1981). *Coping with difficult people.* Garden City, NY: Anchor Books/Doubleday.

Brophy, S.F. (1974). The RN problem: Returning to active practice. *Journal of Nursing Administration*, 4(9&10), 45–48.

Bushong, N.V.K., & Simms, S. (1979). Externship: A way to bridge the gap. *Supervisor Nurse*, 10(6), 14–22.

Cantor, M.M. (1978). *Achieving nursing care standards: Internal & external.* Wakefield, MA: Nursing Resources.

Caruth, D. (1983). How to delegate successfully. *Supervisory Management*, 28(2), 36–42.

Caruth, D., & Middlebrook, B. (1981). How to make a better decision. *Supervisory Management*, 26(7), 12–17.

Chagares, R.I. (1980). The nurse internship program revisited. *Supervisor Nurse*, 11(11), 22–24.

Chatham, M.A. (1979). Discrepancies in learning needs assessments: Whose needs are being assessed? *Journal of Continuing Education in Nursing*, 10(5), 18–22.

Chickerella, B.G., & Lutz, W.J. (1981). Professional nurturance: Preceptorships for undergraduate nursing students. *American Journal of Nursing*, 81(1), 107–109.

Clark, C.C. (1980). Burnout: Assessment and intervention. *Journal of Nursing Administration*, 10(9), 39–43.

Clark, C.C. (1979). *The nurse as continuing educator.* New York: Springer.

Clark, K.M., & Dickson, G. (1976). Self-directed and other-directed continuing education: A study of nurses' participation. *Journal of Continuing Education in Nursing*, 7(4), 16–24.

Colavecchio, R., Tescher, B., & Scalzi, C. (1974). A clinical ladder for nursing practice. *Journal of Nursing Administration*, 4(9&10), 54–58.

Conley, V. (1973). *Curriculum and instruction in nursing.* Boston: Little, Brown.

Cooper, S.S. (1982). Methods of teaching revisited: Nursing rounds and bedside clinics. *Journal of Continuing Education in Nursing*, 13(5), 19–21.

Cooper, S.S. (1980). *Self directed learning in nursing.* Wakefield, MA: Nursing Resources.

Cronin-Stubbs, D., & Mathews, J. (1982). A clinical performance evaluation tool for a process oriented nursing curriculum. *Nurse Educator*, 7(4), 24–29.

Curran, C.L. (1977). What kind of continuing education? *Supervisor Nurse*, 8(7), 72–75.

Davis, A.J. (1963). The skills of communication. *American Journal of Nursing*, 63(1), 66–70.

Dear, M.R., Celentano, D.D., Weisman, C.S., & Keen, M.F. (1982). Evaluating a hospital nursing internship. *Journal of Nursing Administration*, 12(11), 16–20.

Del Bueno, D.J. (1982). Is your inservice program a waste of money? *RN*, 45(5), 24q, 24s–t.

Dell, M.S., & Griffith, E. (1977). A preceptor program for nurses' clinical orientation. *Journal of Nursing Administration*, 7(1), 37–38.

Diffie-Couch, P. (1983). How to give feedback. *Supervisory Management*, 28(8), 27–31.

Donovan, L. (1980). Can you really make more as a grocery clerk? Nursing incomes survey: Part III. *RN*, 43(50), 51–54, 66.

Donovan, L. (1980). The shortage. *RN*, *43*(6), 21–27.

Douglass, M.E., & Douglass, D.N. (1980). *Manage your time, manage your work, manage yourself.* New York: AMACOM.

Drake, J.D. (1982). *Interviewing for managers* (rev. ed.). New York: AMACOM.

Drucker, P.F. (1973). *Management: Tasks, responsibilities, practices.* New York: Harper & Row.

Dunn, R., Debello, T., Brennan, P., Krimensky, J., & Murrain, P. (1981). Learning style researchers define differences differently. *Educational Leadership*, *38*(5), 372–375.

Engstrom, T.W., & MacKenzie, R.A. (1967). *Managing your time.* Grand Rapids, MI: Zondervan.

Everson, S., Panoc, K., Pratt, P., & King, A.M. (1981). Precepting as an entry method for newly hired staff. *Journal of Continuing Education in Nursing*, *12*(6), 22–26.

Fairbanks, J. (1980). Primary nursing: What's so exciting about it? *Nursing*, *10*(11), 55–57.

Fast, J. (1970). *Body language.* New York: Simon & Schuster.

Fear, R.A. (1978). *The evaluation interview* (rev. 2nd ed.). New York: McGraw-Hill.

Felts, B. (1975). The change in nurse education. *Hospital Forum*, *18*(2), 9–10, 20.

Ferris, L. (1980). Cardiac preceptor model: Access to learning by nurses in rural communities. *Journal of Continuing Education in Nursing*, *11*(1), 19–23.

Fralic, M.V. (1980). Nursing shortage: Coping today and planning for tomorrow. *Hospitals*, *54*(9), 65–67.

Friedman, W.H., Ganong, J.M., & Ganong, W.L. (1979). Workshopping. *Nurse Educator*, *4*(6), 19–22.

Friesen, L., & Conahan, B.J. (1980). A clinical preceptor program: Strategy for new graduate orientation. *Journal of Nursing Administration*, *10*(4), 18–23.

Ganong, J.M., & Ganong, W.L. (1980). *Nursing management* (2nd ed.). Rockville, MD: Aspen Systems.

Garity, J. (1983). Developing head nurses: One hospital's solution. *Nurse Educator*, *9*(3), 38–42.

Gessner, B.A. (1979). McClusky's concept of margin. *Journal of Continuing Education in Nursing*, *10*(2), 39–44.

Getting fed up? (1981). *RN*, *44*(1), 18–25.

Ghiglieri, S., Woods, S.A., & Moyer, K. (1983). Toward a competency based safe practice. *Nursing Management*, *14*(3), 16–19.

Gibb, J.R. (1961). Defensive communication. *Journal of Communication*, *11*(3), 141–148.

Goldfinch, J. (1982). Training supervisors through behavior modeling. *Hospital Topics*, *60*(3), 33–34.

Goodale, J.G. (1981). The neglected art of interviewing. *Supervisory Management*, *26*(7), 2–11.

Grandbouche, A. (1982). It's time to put a proper price on nursing. *RN*, *45*(5), 83–84.

Granick, S., & Patterson, R. (1971). *Human aging II: An eleven year follow-up.* (DHEW Publication No. HSM 71-9037). Washington, DC: U.S. Government Printing Office. In H.C. Moidel, E.C. Giblin, & B.M. Wagner, (Eds.). (1976). *Nursing care of the patient with medical-surgical disorders* (2nd ed.). New York: McGraw-Hill.

Halatin, T.J., & Knotts, R.E. (1982). Becoming a mentor: Are the risks worth the rewards? *Supervisory Management*, *27*(2), 27–29.

Hall, E.T. (1969). *The hidden dimension.* Garden City, NY: Anchor Books/Doubleday.

Hallas, G.G. (1980). Why nurses are giving it up. *RN*, *42*(7), 17–21.

Hammerstad, S.M., Johnson, S.H., & Land, L.V. (1977). New graduate orientation program. *Journal of Continuing Education in Nursing*, *8*(5), 5–11.

Hartin, J.M. (1983). Nursing apprenticeship. *Nursing Management*, *14*(3), 28–29.

Hathaway, D. (1981). Rooting out reality shock. *Journal of Practical Nursing*, *31*(11 & 12), 42–44.

Hathaway, D. (1980). When the honeymoon is over: Dealing with the real world of nursing. *Journal of Practical Nursing*, *30*(7), 32–33, 41–42.

Havighurst, R.J., & Orr, B. (1956). *Adult education and adult needs*. Chicago: Center for the Study of Liberal Education for Adults.

Haynor, P. (1978). Career ladder—Back to the bedside. *Supervisor Nurse*, *9*(2), 33–36.

Helmuth, M.R., & Guberski, T.D. (1980). Preparation for the preceptor role. *Nursing Outlook*, *28*(1), 36–39.

Hermann, W.J. (1982). Developing job descriptions. *Medical Group Management*, 29(3), 44–48.

Hersey, P., & Blanchard, K. (1982). *Management of organizational behavior: Utilizing human resources* (4th ed.). Englewood Cliffs, NJ: Prentice-Hall.

Herzberg, F. (1968). One more time: How do you motivate employees? *Harvard Business Review* *46*(1), 53–62.

Hildebrand, M. (1973). The character and skills of the effective professor. Columbus: Ohio State University Press, pp. 41–50.

Hohman, J. (1979). Nurse mentor system cuts costs, boosts quality of patient care. *Hospitals*, 53(1), 93–94; 101.

Ingalls, J.D., & Arceri, J.M. (1972). *A trainer's guide to androgogy*. Waltham, MA: Data Education.

Januarygari, M., & Duffy, P. (1980). Contracting with patients in day to day practice. *American Journal of Nursing*, *80*(3), 451–455.

Jehring, J.J. (1972). Motivational problems in the modern hospital. *Journal of Nursing Administration*, *1*(11 & 12), 35–41.

Johnson, W. (1980). Supply and demand for registered nurses. *Nursing and Health Care*, *1*(2), 73–79; 112.

Jones, P., & Oertel, W. (1977). Developing patient teaching objectives and techniques: A self instructional program. *Nurse Educator*, *2*(5), 3–18.

Kelly, L.Y. (1978). Power guide—The mentor relationship. *Nursing Outlook*, *26*(5), 339.

Kirk, R. (1981). *Nursing management tools*. Boston: Little, Brown.

Knauss, P.J. (1980). Staff nurse preceptorship: An experiment for graduate nurse orientation. *Journal of Continuing Education in Nursing*, *11*(5), 44–46.

Knowles, M. (1973). *The adult learner: A neglected species*. Houston: Gulf Publishing.

Knowles, M. (1970). *The modern practice of adult education*. New York: Association Press.

Kolb, D.A. (1976a). *Learning style inventory: Self scoring test and interpretation booklet*. Boston: McBer and Company.

Kolb, D.A. (1976b). Learning style inventory: Technical manual. Boston: McBer and Company.

Kolb, D.A., & Boyatizes, A. (1974). Goal setting and self directed behavior. In D.A. Kolb, I. Rubin, & J. McIntyre, *Organizational psychology: A book of readings* (2nd ed.). Englewood Cliffs, NJ: Prentice-Hall.

Kolb, D.A., Rubin, I., & McIntyre, J. (1974). *Organizational psychology: A book of readings* (2nd ed.). Englewood Cliffs, NJ: Prentice-Hall.

Kolb, D.A., Rubin, I., & McIntyre, J. (1974). *Organizational psychology: An experiential approach*. Englewood Cliffs, NJ: Prentice-Hall.

Kotler, P. (1972). *Marketing management: Analysis, planning and control* (2nd ed.). Englewood Cliffs, NJ: Prentice-Hall.

Kramer, M. (1974). *Reality shock: Why nurses leave nursing*. St. Louis: Mosby.

Krathwohl, D.R., Bloom, B.S., & Masia, B. (1964). *Taxonomy of educational objectives: The classification of educational goals. Handbook II: Affective Domain*. New York: David McKay.

Kron, T. (1967). *Communication in nursing*. Philadelphia: Saunders.

Lakin, A. (1973). *How to get control of your time and your life*. New York: New American Library.

Lancaster, J. (1980). *Adult psychiatric nursing*. Garden City, NY: Medical Examination Co.

Lavandero, R. (1981). Nurse burnout: What can we learn? *Journal of Nursing Administration, 11*(11 & 12), 17–23.

Lawless, D.J. (1972). *Effective management: Social psychological approach*. Englewood Cliffs, NJ: Prentice-Hall.

Lea, D., & Leibowitz, Z.B. (1983). A mentor: Would you know one if you saw one? *Supervisory Management, 27*(4), 33–35.

Le Boeuf, M. (1979). *Working smart: How to accomplish more in half the time*. New York: McGraw-Hill.

Le Duc, S.S. (1979). We've been put down long enough. *RN, 42*(12), 67–68, 70.

Lee, A. (1979). Still the handmaiden. *RN, 43*(12), 21–30.

Levine, E. (1980). Let's talk: Breaking down barriers to effective communication. *Supervisory Management, 25*(6), 2–13.

Lewison, D., & Gibbons, L.K. (1980). Nursing internships: A comprehensive review of the literature. *Journal of Continuing Education in Nursing, 11*(2), 32–38.

Limon, S., Bargagliotti, L.A., & Spencer, J.B. (1980). Providing preceptors for nursing students: What questions should you ask? *Journal of Nursing Administration, 12*(6), 16–19.

Limon, S., Bargagliotti, L.A., & Spencer, J.B. (1981). Who precepts the preceptor? *Nursing & Health Care, 2*(3), 453–436.

Lorig, K. (1977). An overview of needs assessment tools for continuing education. *Nurse Educator, 2*(2), 12–16.

Lucke, Z. (1979). Pitfalls in preceptorship. *Nursing Administration Quarterly, 4*(1), 29.

MacKenzie, R.A. (1973, December 3). How to make the most of your time. *U.S. News and World Report*, pp. 45–48, 53–54.

Mager, R.F. (1975). *Preparing educational objectives* (2nd ed.). Belmont, CA: Fearon Pitman.

Mahr, D.R. (1979). RN preceptors: Do they help students in the OR? *AORN, 30*(4), 724–730.

Maraldo, P.J. (1977). Better nursing care through preceptorships. *RN, 40*(3), 69–71.

Martel, G.D., & Edmunds, M.W. (1972). Nurse internship program in Chicago. *American Journal of Nursing, 72*(5), 940–943.

Martin, P.D. (1976). The graduate nurse transition program. *Supervisor Nurse, 7*(12), 18, 20, 22.

Maslow, A.H. (1968). *Toward a psychology of being* (2nd ed.). New York: Van Nostrand Reinhold.

Massey, M. (1979). *The people puzzle: Understanding yourself and others*. Reston, VA: Reston Publishing.

Mauly, G. (1968). *Psychology for effective teaching* (2nd ed.). New York: Holt, Rinehart & Winston.

May, L. (1980). Clinical preceptors for new nurses. *American Journal of Nursing, 80*(10), 1824–1826.

McAlindon, H.R. (1980). Toward a more creative you: The actualizing climate. *Supervisory Management, 25*(4), 35–40.

McCay, J.T. (1959). *The management of time*. Englewood Cliffs, NJ: Prentice-Hall.

McConnell, C.R. (1982). *The effective health care supervisor*. Rockville, MD: Aspen Systems.

McConnell, E.A. (1981). How close are you to burnout? *RN*, *44*(5), 29–33.

McElroy, A.M. (1982). Burnout—A review of the literature with application to cancer nursing. *Cancer Nursing*, *5*(3), 211–217.

McGrath, B.J., & Koewing, J.R. (1978). A clinical preceptorship for new graduate nurses. *Journal of Nursing Administration*, *8*(3), 12–18.

McGregor, D. (1960). *The human side of enterprise*. New York: McGraw-Hill.

McLagan, P.A. (1978). *Helping others learn: Designing programs for adults*. Reading, MA: Addison-Wesley.

McNeil, E.B., & Rubin, Z. (1977). *The psychology of being human* (2nd ed.). San Francisco: Canfield Press.

Miller, S. (1978). Letter from a new graduate. *American Journal of Nursing*, *78*(10), 1688.

Miller, R. (1975). Career ladder: A problem solving device. *Journal of Nursing Administration*, *7*(6), 27–29.

Minor, M.A., & Thompson, L. (1981). Nurse internship program based on nursing process. *Supervisor Nurse*, *12*(1), 28–31.

Moraldo, P.J. (1977). Better nursing care through preceptorships. *RN*, *40*(3), 69–71.

Moran, V. (1977). Study of comparison of independent learning activities vs. attendance at staff development by staff nurses. *Journal of Continuing Education in Nursing*, *8*(3), 14–21.

Moyer, M.G., & Mann, J.K. (1979). A preceptor program of orientation within the critical care area. *Heart and Lung*, *8*(3), 530–534.

Muniz, P., & Chasnoff, R. (1982). Counseling the marginal performer. *Supervisory Management*, *27*(5), 2–14.

Munn, H.E., Jr. (1975). Developing and improving your communication skills. *Hospital Topics*, *53*(6), 40–43.

Munn, H.E., Jr. (1980). *The nurse's communication handbook*. Rockville, MD: Aspen Systems.

Murphy, J. (1979). The first hour: Creating a learning environment. *Journal of Continuing Education in Nursing*, *10*(5), 42–46.

Murray, J.E. (1964). *Motivation and emotion*. Englewood Cliffs, NJ: Prentice-Hall.

Murray, R., & Zentner, J. (1975). *Nursing concepts for health promotion*. Englewood Cliffs, NJ: Prentice-Hall.

Newstrom, J.W., & Scannel, E.E. (1980). *Games trainers play: Experiential learning exercises*. New York: McGraw-Hill.

Nordmark, M.T., & Rohweder, A.W. (1967). *Scientific foundations of nursing*. Philadelphia: Lippincott.

Norman, J. (1978). The clinical specialist as performance appraiser. *Supervisor Nurse*, *9*(7), 62–64.

Norris, C.G. (1980). Characteristics of the adult learner and extended higher education for registered nurses. *Nursing & Health Care*, *1*(2), 87–93.

The nurse shortage: There's a long road ahead. (1980). *Hospitals*, *54*(9), 63–64.

O'Brien, A. (1982). Choosing the role in staff development that's best for you. *AORN*, *35*(7), 1262–1267.

O'Connor, A.B. (1982). Staff development: The problems of motivation. *Journal of Continuing Education in Nursing*, *13*(2), 10–14.

Oermann, M. (1977). Diagnostic supervision. *Supervisor Nurse*, *8*(11), 9–14.

Olson, R.F. (1980). *Managing the interview*. New York: Wiley.

Pardue, S.F. (1983). The who-what-why of mentor teacher/graduate student relationships. *Journal of Nursing Education*, 22(1), 32–37.

Parsons, J. (1976). A new approach to group learning. *Journal of Continuing Education in Nursing*, 7(4), 5–9.

Patrick, P. (1979). Burnout: Job hazard for health workers. *Hospitals*, 87–88, 90.

Patton, D., Grace, A., & Roca, J. (1981). Implementation of the preceptor concepts: Adaptation to high stress climate. *Journal of Continuing Education in Nursing*, 12(5), 27–31.

Phegley, D. (1976). Designing the nursing management program through objective needs survey. *Supervisor Nurse*, 7(11), 28–32.

Pillette, P.C. (1978). The mentor relationship (letter). *Nursing Outlook*, 26(8), 473.

Pines, A.M., & Aronson, E. (1981). *Burnout: From tedium to personal growth*. New York: Free Press.

Popliel, E.S. (1977). *Nursing and the process of continuing education* (2nd ed.). St. Louis: Mosby.

Porter-O'Grady, T. (1982). What motivation isn't. *Nursing Management*, 13(12), 27–30.

Predd, C.S. (1982). Setting priorities: How to stay efficient in hectic nursing stations. *Nursing Life*, 2(3), 50–51.

Puetz, B.E., & Peters, F.L. (1981). *Continuing education for nurses: A guide to effective programs*. Rockville, MD: Aspen Systems.

Rationale for a nurse manager preceptorship (Review of *A Management Preceptorship Program* by Joan Garity). (1982). *Nurse Educator*, 7(6), 21–22.

Redman, B.K. (1976). *The process of patient teaching in nursing* (3rd ed.). St. Louis: Mosby.

Reilly, D.E. (1978). *Teaching and evaluating the affective domain in nursing programs*. Thorofare, NJ: Slack.

Reynolds, M.L. (1980). A classification system for RNs. *Supervisor Nurse*, 11(10), 26–28.

Roell, S.M. (1981). Nurse-intern programs: How they're working. *Journal of Nursing Administration*, 11(10), 33–36.

Rowland, H.S., & Rowland, B.L. (1980). *Nursing administration handbook*. Rockville, MD: Aspen Systems.

Sa'di, [Gulistan]. (1970). In R.T. Tripp (Ed.), *The International Thesaurus of Quotations* (James Ross, Trans.). New York: Crowell. (Original quotation 1258).

Sanders, M.M. (1980). Stressed or burned out? *The Canadian Nurse*, 76(10), 30–33.

Sandroff, R. (1980). The shortage: How it's changing nursing. *RN*, 43(11), 55–59, 86, 88, 90.

Sanford, N.D. (1989). Teaching strategies for inservice and staff development instructors. *Journal of Continuing Education in Nursing*, 10(6), 5–10.

Schmalenberg, C., & Kramer, M. (1979). *Coping with reality shock: The voices of experience*. Wakefield, MA: Nursing Resources.

Schoen, D.C. (1979). Lifelong learning: How some participants see it. *Journal of Continuing Education in Nursing*, 10(2), 3–16.

Schoor, T. (1979). Mentorship remembered (editorial). *American Journal of Nursing*, 79(1), 65.

Schweer, J.E., & Gebbie, K.M. (1976). *Creative teaching in clinical nursing* (3rd ed.). St. Louis: Mosby.

Scully, R. (1983). The staff educator as process consultant. *Nurse Educator*, 8(2), 39–42.

Selg, M.J., & Morrow, K.L. (1981). *Graduate nurse residency program: Plan IV*. Everett, WA: Providence Hospital.

Seltiz, C., Wrightsman, L.S., & Cook, S.W. (1976). *Research methods in social relations* (3rd ed.). New York: Holt, Rinehart & Winston.

Selye, H. (1976). *Stress in health and disease*. London: Butterworth.

Seven "sins of supervision" that cancel out cooperation. (1975). *The Manager's Bulletin*, 2(5), 1. (Burbank, CA: St. Joseph Medical Center).

Seybolt, J.W., & Walker, D.D. (1980). Attitude survey proves to be a powerful tool for reversing turnover. *Hospitals*, 54(9), 77–80.

Shaw, M., & Phillips, S. (1982, April 16). Kolb's cognitive learning model. Paper presented at the meeting of the American Society of Health Education and Training, Seattle, WA.

Sheehy, G. (1976). *Passages: Predictable crises of adult life*. New York: Dutton.

Shields, M. (1974). An evaluation model for service programs. *Nursing Outlook*, 22(7), 448–451.

Shipp, T. (1981). Cost benefit analysis for continuing education. *Journal of Continuing Education in Nursing*, 12(4), 6–14.

Smith, M., & Wing, J. (1983). Five steps to improving employee performance. *Supervisory Management*, 28(4), 36–42.

Smoyak, S.A. (1978). Teaching as coaching. *Nursing Outlook*, 26(6), 361–363.

Sondak, A. (1980). The importance of knowing your employees' needs. *Supervisory Management*, 25(5), 13–18.

Sonnen, B.E. (1980). Bloom's theory of school learning. *Journal of Continuing Education in Nursing*, 12(1), 38–41.

Sonnen, B.E. (1980). Thinking about learning: Because I am a learner, what questions should I ask myself as a facilitator? *Journal of Continuing Education in Nursing*, 11(4), 50–56.

Sovie, M. (1980). The role of staff development in hospital cost control. *Nurse Educator*, 5(6), 25–28.

Stanton, E.S. (1974). Do yourself a favor—Pick the right person for the job. *Supervisory Management*, 19(3), 32–40.

Stein, L.S. (1971). The individual curriculum and nursing leadership. *Journal of Continuing Education in Nursing*, 2(6), 7–13.

Steines, P.A. (1982). Be positive not punitive. *Nursing Management*, 13(3), 29–32.

Stevens, B.J. (1976). *First line patient care management*. Wakefield, MA: Nursing Resources.

Stewart, N. (1978). *The effective woman manager*. New York: Wiley.

Storlie, F. (1979). Burnout: The elaboration of a concept. *American Journal of Nursing*, 79(12), 2108–2111.

Stress: In depth. (1982). *Bostonia*, 56(4 & 5), 3, 9–66.

Stritter, F.T., Hain, J.D., & Grimes, D.A. (1975). Clinical teaching reexamined. *Journal of Medical Education*, 50(9), 876–882.

Tarnow, K.G. (1979). Working with adult learners. *Nurse Educator*, 4(5), 34–40.

Tenzer, I.E. (1977). Nursing students learn OR skills. *AORN Journal*, 26(1), 62–68.

Thomas, C. (1980). Understanding the new nurse. *Supervisor Nurse*, 11(1), 46–47.

Thorpe, R. (1980). Cross training program for nurses: Solution to a staffing problem. *Supervisor Nurse*, 11(10), 66–67.

Thorpe, R. (1981). Sabotage in nursing. *Supervisor Nurse*, 12(5), 24–25.

Tobin, H.M., Hull, P.K., & Yoder Wise, P.S. (1979). *The process of staff development* (2nd ed.). St. Louis: Mosby.

Troisi, A.M. (1980). Softening the blow of "you're fired." *Supervisory Management*, 25(6), 14–19.

Turnbull, E. (1983). Rewards in nursing: The case of nurse preceptors. *Journal of Nursing Administration*, 13(1), 10–12.

Uris, A. (1968). *Mastery of management.* Homewood, IL: Dow Jones Irwin.

Van Maanen, J. (Ed.). (1977). *Organizational careers: Some new perspectives.* New York: Wiley.

Verduin, J.R., Jr., Miller, H.G., & Greer, C.E. (1977). *Adults teaching adults.* Austin, TX: Learning Concepts.

Vroom V.H., & Yetten, P.W. (1973). *Leadership and decision making.* Pittsburgh: University of Pittsburgh Press.

Wandelt, M.A., & Stewart, D.S. (1975). *Slater nursing competencies rating scale.* New York: Appleton-Century-Crofts.

Washington State Practical Nurse Practice Act, RCW 18.78.

Webster's seventh new collegiate dictionary. (1967). Springfield, MA: G. & C. Merriam.

Weisgerber, R.A. (1971). *Perspectives in individualized learning.* Itasca, IL: Peacock.

Weiss, W.H. (1983). *The supervisor's problem solver.* New York: AMACOM.

White, C.H. (1980). Where have all the nurses gone—and why? *Hospitals*, 54(9), 68–71.

Wimbush, F.B. (1983). Nurse burnout: Its effect on patient care. *Nursing Management*, 14(1), 55–57.

Yoder Wise, P.S. (1979). Barriers (or enhancers) to adult education. *Journal of Continuing Education in Nursing*, 10(6), 11–16.

Yoder Wise, P.S. (1979). Preparing budgets for inservice educators. *Journal of Continuing Education in Nursing*, 10(6), 17–23.

Yunek, M. (1980). Self assessment of learning needs: A tool to assist nurses in self directed learning. *Journal of Continuing Education in Nursing*, 11(5), 30–33.

Index

Note: Page numbers appearing in *italics* indicate artwork.

person performing, 120
by persons in helping roles, 121
purpose of, 119
questionnaires in, 123
by self, 120-121
suggestion boxes in, 124
techniques for, 121-124
tests in, 122
and novice. *See* Novice(s) and
  preceptor
one-way communication from,
  noncommunication with novice
  due to, 82-83
performance guidelines for, *43*
pool of, for preceptor program, 20-21
in preliminary program, 30
problems of, common, 75-86
qualifications for, 53-54
recruitment of, in program
  improvement and expansion,
  108-110
remuneration for, in budget
  preparation, 39
replacement of, in program
  improvement and expansion,
  108-110
responsibilities of, *15*
role of, 5-7, 113-114
selection of, criteria for, 207
self-care of, 193-205
  stress management in, 200-204
    See also Stress
  time management in, 193-200
    See also Time, management of,
    by preceptors
and staff, relationship between, 118
as supervisors, 169-178
  See also Supervision
too busy, noncommunication with
  novice due to, 82
workshop for example of, 251-253
Preceptor program(s)
appropriateness of, 17-18
coordination of, 20
decision on establishment of,
  21-22

developing and managing, 1-110
evaluation of, 89-104
  See also Evaluation of preceptor
  program
expansion of, 108
  preceptor recruitment and
  replacement in, 108-110
feasibility of, 19-22
flexibility in, 21
funding for, 21
in graduate nurse residency,
  evaluation forms for, 241-245
implementation of, 61-73
  novice selection in, 68-69
  pairing preceptor and novice in,
  69-70
  piloting in, 70-72
  preceptor development in, 61-68
    See also Preceptor(s),
    development of
improvement of, 105-108
  goals in, 107-108
  needs for, assessment of, 106-107
  objectives in, 107-108
  preceptor recruitment and
  replacement for, 108-110
  prioritization in, 107
  reasons for, 105-106
inappropriateness for, 18-19
leadership for, 19
need for, 17-22
objectives of, overall, in preliminary
  program draft, 34
personnel for, finding, 49-59
  See also Personnel
planning, 23-47
  exploration phase of, 23-34
    See also Exploration phase of
    preceptor program planning
  preparation phase of, 35-47
    See also Preparation phase of
    preceptor program planning
preceptor pool for, 20-21
purpose of, in preliminary program
  draft, 29
support for, 19-20